Praise for

The Whole Body Reset

"Our bodies change with age, and the way we eat needs to change in response. *The Whole Body Reset* is the first program written specifically for people at midlife who want to stay lean, active, and strong for decades to come."

—Sanjay Gupta, MD, chief medical correspondent for CNN,
#1 *New York Times* bestselling author of *Keep Sharp*,
and associate professor of neurosurgery at
Emory University School of Medicine

"Gaining weight at midlife is common, but it's not inevitable. *The Whole Body Reset* is a plan that can not only stop but even reverse age-related weight gain and muscle loss. The best part is that it's simple, and it works!"

—Ian K. Smith, MD, *New York Times* bestselling
author of *FAST Burn* and former member of the
President's Council on Sports, Fitness & Nutrition

"Finally, a nutrition program I would recommend to family and friends in their forties, fifties, and beyond. It's new, crucial information that can change your life."

—Travis Stork, MD, Emmy-nominated former cohost of
The Doctors and *New York Times* bestselling author of
The Lean Belly Prescription

"As a weight-loss coach for nearly two decades, I couldn't possibly be more excited about *The Whole Body Reset*! I've encountered a debilitated, 'it's-just-not-going-to-work-at-my-age' mindset in middle-aged plus clients more times than I can count. To FINALLY have a concrete resource full of sensible strategies that promote muscle gain and overall health, backed by scientific evidence, is a game changer."

—Devin Alexander, celebrity chef, weight-loss coach, and *New York Times* bestselling author of The Biggest Loser Cookbook series

"It is never too late to change your life, as long as you have smart, science-driven information at your fingertips. *The Whole Body Reset* is a breakthrough program that gives you the tools you need to turn back the clock and reclaim your physique, your health, and your life."

—Marco Borges, nutritionist, exercise physiologist, and founder of 22 Days Nutrition

"In smart, easy-to-digest language, *The Whole Body Reset* explains how simple tweaks to our daily eating habits can make our bodies respond as though they are twenty or thirty years younger."

—Mark Hyman, MD, Pritzker Foundation Chair in Functional Medicine, Cleveland Clinic, and *New York Times* bestselling author of *The Pegan Diet*

"As I approached fifty, I noticed my body was changing. *The Whole Body Reset* explains how and why this happens, and what to do to get back into ideal physical shape."

—Jorge Cruise, celebrity personal trainer, nutritionist, and *New York Times* bestselling author of *The Belly Fat Cure*

"Finally, an easy-to-follow plan that means getting older can be the best time of your life. Thank you, Stephen and Heidi, for turning me on to protein timing!"

—Meredith Vieira, journalist and former host of
Today and *The View*

"The book's strength is its wealth of helpful tools: there's a guide to making sense of labels, shopping list suggestions, and a seven-day sample menu planner with entrées from such restaurants as Buffalo Wild Wings and Chipotle. Readers looking for new health tricks to replace strategies that no longer work will find this a resource worth returning to."

—*Publishers Weekly*

ALSO BY STEPHEN PERRINE

The New American Diet
The Men's Health Diet
The Women's Health Diet
Pretty Intense (with Danica Patrick)
Zero Sugar Diet (with David Zinczenko)

ALSO BY HEIDI SKOLNIK

Nutrient Timing for Peak Performance
Grill Yourself Skinny
The Reverse Diet (with Tricia Cunningham)

THE
WHOLE
BODY
RESET

Your Weight-Loss Plan for a *Flat Belly*,
Optimum Health, and a *Body You'll Love*
— at Midlife and Beyond —

STEPHEN PERRINE
WITH HEIDI SKOLNIK

Simon & Schuster Paperbacks

NEW YORK   LONDON   TORONTO
SYDNEY   NEW DELHI

Simon & Schuster Paperbacks
An Imprint of Simon & Schuster, Inc.
1230 Avenue of the Americas
New York, NY 10020

A range of AARP print and e-books are available at AARP's online bookstore, aarp.org/bookstore, and through local and online bookstores.

First Simon & Schuster trade paperback edition December 2023

SIMON & SCHUSTER PAPERBACKS and colophon are registered trademarks of Simon & Schuster, Inc.

For information about special discounts for bulk purchases, please contact Simon & Schuster Special Sales at 1-866-506-1949 or business@simonandschuster.com.

The Simon & Schuster Speakers Bureau can bring authors to your live event. For more information or to book an event, contact the Simon & Schuster Speakers Bureau at 1-866-248-3049 or visit our website at www.simonspeakers.com.

Interior design by Paul Dippolito

Printed and bound by CPI Group (UK) Ltd, Croydon CR0 4YY

10 9 8 7 6 5 4 3 2 1

Library of Congress Cataloging-in-Publication Data

Names: Perrine, Stephen, author. | Skolnik, Heidi, 1961– author.
Title: The whole body reset : your weight-loss plan for a flat belly, optimum health, and a body you'll love— at midlife and beyond / Stephen Perrine, AARP Executive Editor with Heidi Skolnik.
Description: First Simon & Schuster hardcover edition. | New York : Simon & Schuster, 2022. | Includes index.
Identifiers: LCCN 2021042305 | ISBN 9781982160128 (hardcover) | ISBN 9781982160173 (ebook)
Subjects: LCSH: Reducing diets. | Nutrition. | Health.
Classification: LCC RM222.2 P43467 2022 | DDC 613.2/5—dc23/eng/20211014
LC record available at https://lccn.loc.gov/2021042305

ISBN 978-1-9821-6012-8
ISBN 978-1-6680-8249-2 (pbk)
ISBN 978-1-9821-6017-3 (ebook)

Contents

CONTENTS

The Whole Body Reset Advisory Board

Errol Green, RPh, MD, FACEP, Emergency Medicine, Tufts Medical Center, Boston, MA (retired), and AARP medical advisor

Jordan Metzl, MD, sports medicine physician, Hospital for Special Surgery

Steven Nissen, MD, chairman of the Department of Cardiovascular Medicine, Cleveland Clinic, and past president of the American College of Cardiology

Douglas Paddon-Jones, PhD, FACSM, Sheridan Lorenz Distinguished Professor in Aging and Health, Department of Nutrition and Metabolism, School of Health Professions, University of Texas Medical Branch

Pamela Peeke, MD, MPII, FACP, FACSM, Pew Foundation Scholar in Nutrition and Metabolism, assistant professor of medicine, University of Maryland, and Director of the Peeke Performance Center for Healthy Living

Adriana Perez, PhD, ANP-BC, FAAN, associate professor of nursing, University of Pennsylvania School of Nursing

Introduction:
A Flat Belly at 50+

You don't have to gain weight as you age.

All the negatives we associate with age fifty and beyond—an expanding midsection, softer muscles, and general physical decline?

They aren't inevitable.

They're avoidable.

Indeed, they're even reversible.

And yet . . .

The vast majority of us struggle with weight gain in middle age. The standard weight-loss tricks that may have worked in our thirties and forties no longer keep the weight off. We may be eating just as healthfully and exercising just as much, but we're still gaining weight, seemingly faster than ever before. Why?

This book answers that question. And it lays out the simple, proven, and effective program that can reverse age-related weight gain and muscle loss, flatten your belly, and slash your risk of disability, disease, and mental and physical decline.

This isn't a fad diet.

This isn't like anything you've ever read before.

This is the Whole Body Reset.

"I Used to Be Thin . . ."

Wherever you're sitting right now, take a moment to glance down.

See your belly? It's larger than it once was, isn't it?

Belly fat evokes a lot of feelings. It's easy to take this growing expanse, this "middle-age spread," as a personal affront. It's right there in front of us, all the time, and it just won't seem to go away. In fact, if anything, it keeps getting bigger. No matter how many exercise programs we've tried, how many diets we've attempted, how many supplements or "superfoods" we've eaten, belly fat is as stubborn as a tired three-year-old—it won't be moved by any amount of logic, any degree of bargaining or begging. In fact, between our twenties and our sixties, men on average experience a more than 200 percent increase in visceral fat—that's the fat that lies deep in our bellies, hanging around our internal organs like rock-star groupies. Women see a 400 percent increase in this type of fat.

Maybe, we tell ourselves, our belly fat is a sign that we've failed.

Or maybe, it's just a sign that we're getting old.

If you've ever felt that way, well, I'm right there with you.

For most of my life, managing my weight was easy. In fact, weight loss was practically my career: I've researched, written about, and followed just about every diet trend of the past several decades. I've broken gluten-free bread with tennis champ Novak Djokovic and broken a sweat alongside race car driver Danica Patrick. I've followed Paleo, low-fat, low-carb, vegetarian, vegan, and anti-obesogenic diet plans. I've intermittent-fasted, I've cleansed, I've gone organic and sugar-free. I spent nearly two decades working at *Men's Health,* where we practically invented the word "abs." And for most of that time, I edited the highly successful Eat This, Not That! franchise, first as a food column, then as a book series, and then as its own magazine and website. I've overseen more than two dozen *New York Times* bestsellers in the diet and nutrition field as an author, editor, or publisher.

In other words, if you can eat it, I've probably written a book on it.

Then, a few years ago, two things happened. First, I turned fifty. Then I joined the staff of AARP.

As executive editor, I oversee health and wellness coverage for *AARP The Magazine* and the *AARP Bulletin*. When our nearly 38 million members write in with their health and fitness concerns, I'm the guy whose in-box gets flooded. And among our members, one worry pops up over and over: *"I used to be thin. Now I'm overweight. And there doesn't seem to be anything I can do about it."*

That's how I felt, too. I was eating the same way I always had, enjoying the same healthy, balanced diet that had kept me in size 32 pants well into my forties. But my old clothes weren't fitting anymore, my belly was getting larger, and my old way of eating and exercising wasn't cutting it.

As a health journalist, I knew that this new front porch was doing more than making me look bad; belly fat is dangerous. Unlike the subcutaneous ("under the skin") fat you can pinch between your fingers, our belly, or visceral, fat sits in our abdominal cavity, coating our major organs. As it grows, it generates inflammatory compounds, substances that have been linked to arteriosclerosis, asthma, autoimmune diseases, Alzheimer's . . . and that's just the As. You can add an increased risk of colon, breast, and prostate cancers, type 2 diabetes, stroke, and heart disease to that list. The emergence of COVID-19 put an even finer point on it, as belly fat's sniveling little sidekick—chronic inflammation—arose as one of the top risk factors for coronavirus complications. Being overweight can even increase your risk of taking a fall or dying in a car accident. Bottom line. If it can kill you, there's a good chance belly fat plays a role.

What I needed was a program designed specifically for someone my age—a smart, easy, effective eating plan for a person at midlife and beyond. So I looked around, and I discovered . . .

There's not much out there for people our age.

For all the countless diet programs that claim to "shred" fat, "melt" our bellies, and "supercharge" our metabolisms, few if any are designed to target the specific needs of people at midlife and beyond. Modern diet and weight-loss programs—including popular programs like the South Beach Diet or Whole30, as well as proven, healthy nutrition plans like the Mediterranean diet—have been developed and targeted to the general public. Despite the significant

---

"I went off blood pressure medicines. My cholesterol is better. And it's fun to shop for clothes again!"

Elizabeth Woodward, age 55, Tigard, Oregon

Dropped 22 pounds on the 12-week test panel and 30 pounds overall

Elizabeth knew she needed to make a healthy change.

"I was up thirty pounds over my ideal weight—meaning the weight I wanted to be at," she says. A former exercise physiologist, Elizabeth was already very active, walking six to eight miles every day and going to the gym regularly. So she knew if she was going to drop those unwanted pounds, it meant changing her diet.

"Knowing what you need to do and actually doing it are two different things," she told us. "Then AARP offered this program. I just said, 'Okay, this is my start date. This is what I'm doing.'" She began by becoming more aware of what she was eating, making sure her portions were sensible, and most important of all, adding protein to her breakfasts every day. And sure enough, not only did the pounds start coming off—she lost twenty-two during the Whole Body Reset twelve-week trial—but they kept coming off, and stayed off, even

changes that occur in our bodies as we age—particularly in our hormonal, structural, and digestive systems—no program existed to address the specific needs of people our age.

Even the U.S. government has left people fifty and older in the lurch. The 2020–2025 *Dietary Guidelines for Americans*—which informs everything from food packaging to agricultural policy— includes specific recommendations for every age category: for toddlers, teens, young adults, and folks in their twenties, thirties,

during the pandemic. Today, she's not only thirty pounds lighter, but she recently tried on her wedding dress—and it fit! "My daughter was really impressed," she says.

So is her doctor: Her healthy HDL cholesterol levels rose, her unhealthy LDL levels dropped, and now both are within the recommended guidelines. "I was even able to go off my blood pressure medicine when I dropped the weight," she says. "My doctor put me back on after my weight plateaued, but at a very low dose."

And she did it all without feeling like she was making sacrifices. "I still have my mocha in the morning; that's what I get up for!" Elizabeth says. "And I love ice cream. I still have it almost every night. I'm just careful about what I eat the rest of the day."

But perhaps most important is how she feels. "My energy levels have definitely increased. My mood improved. And now it's fun to shop for clothes again. I couldn't go to the stores because of COVID, so I've been shopping online, and I find that I'm not returning things like I used to, because the clothes fit better.

"I've always worked remotely, but recently I went into the office and they were like, 'Oh my gosh, what happened to you?' Everyone wanted to know what I did. And I said, 'The Whole Body Reset.'"

and forties, broken out by gender, and carefully curated up to age fifty. But there, the *Dietary Guidelines* drops us like hot potatoes. Indeed, there's just one additional set of guidelines for men and another one for women, and all they say is "51+." As far as the government is concerned, outside of recommending more calcium and vitamin D after age seventy, the daily nutritional goals are the same for a fifty-one-year-old woman and her seventy-five-year-old mom.

Does that seem right to you?

Many experts who study the nutritional needs of people fifty and older believe the current guidelines are so far off, they're potentially unhealthy—a recipe for weight gain. And the most surprising fact of all is that there's plenty of science available to show exactly how we should eat to prevent age-related muscle loss, reverse age-related weight gain, and, most important, preserve our long-term health.

It's called "protein timing."

Protein timing is a way of eating that's deceptively simple but has been shown in study after study to halt age-related weight gain, preserve lean muscle, and turn back the tide of what we've come to think of as "natural" decline.

But the word just isn't getting out.

I set out to change that. I've spent the past four years poring over hundreds of studies, talking to scores of researchers, and crunching numbers and ideas with my coauthor, nutritionist and exercise scientist Heidi Skolnik. Now, backed by the mighty resources of AARP, the guidance of a panel of top health experts, and the enthusiastic participation of AARP staffers, I've built a tested and proven, science-based weight-loss program designed specifically for men and women at midlife and beyond. It's the Whole Body Reset, and it's exactly what we need at this stage in our lives.

A Weight-Loss Plan for the Rest of Us

The Whole Body Reset applies up-to-the-minute weight-loss science—drawing from research primarily conducted not on animals, not on the general public, but on people our age. (Because our bodies are different, and a study of a food's effects on yeast, fruit flies, rodents, or twentysomething athletes is not the same as evidence of its effects on our prime-years physiques.) It reveals how protein timing—eating protein in the proper amounts throughout the day—triggers older bodies to spurn fat gain and hold on to lean muscle tissue. This approach, coupled with plenty of fiber, vitamins and minerals, and healthy fats, can help us not only to reshape our bodies, but to reshape our very lives. It's the foundation of the Whole Body Reset.

"I loved the simplicity of the groupings and the help with serving sizes. The recipes were easy and delicious."

—Beth Daniels, age 57, Silver Spring, Maryland
Dropped 19 pounds on the 12-week test panel

This program isn't low-carb or low-fat, it doesn't require calorie counting or periods of food restriction, and it doesn't eliminate any particular food category. But once you know how to do it, and incorporate it into your daily life, it can strip away as much as nineteen pounds in just twelve weeks—with the vast majority of those pounds coming from pure fat while preserving muscle mass, maintaining metabolism, and positively impacting blood pressure and other critical markers of wellness. It can even significantly reduce your risk of

"This is real food that everyone likes!"

Bill Hawkins, age 64, Birmingham, Alabama

Dropped 10 pounds on the 12-week test panel and 40 pounds overall

Weight control has for years been an issue for Bill, a diabetic. And as a result, he's no stranger to weight-loss plans. "I had done every diet known to man. And it's always a struggle," he says. But he couldn't find one he could stick to.

The problem: Most diets just aren't made for real life. "Many of the diets I've read about are things you can't sustain," he told us. "They're geared for folks of different ages, or for people who have access to weird or uncommon ingredients. I have a family, and most programs require foods that they're just not going to eat."

But the Whole Body Reset is different: "When I saw this, it tied into everything I needed. You want meals that are convenient, that meet your needs. This is real food that everyone likes." The diet was so easy that he lost ten pounds during AARP's initial twelve-week pilot, and another thirty pounds during COVID.

The key to success for Bill has been eating more protein, which has allowed him to reduce simple starches and up the number of fruits and vegetables he consumes, without feeling hungry or deprived. "I feel fulfilled, especially in my lunch and nighttime meals," he says.

As a result, he says his diabetes has become much easier to manage: "I feel tremendously better when my blood sugar is under control, and this diet has helped me do that. I can't cut out medicines, but I can drastically reduce the number of times I have to go to the doctor. And I can point to better sleep, which has helped."

many of the chronic diseases of aging, enhancing the overall health of both your body and your brain.

And the Whole Body Reset is easy.

❏ We can eat what we want: There's no weird science that says we can't eat certain food groups like beans, or tomatoes, or bread, or milk, or whatever it is we crave. This plan isn't low-carb, or low-fat, or ketogenic. No foods are required, no foods are off-limits. There are no calorie-counting charts to follow or measurements to take. Nor does the Whole Body Reset require you to eat foods that don't fit your lifestyle or suit your body—whether you're gluten free, vegetarian or vegan, or simply hate eggplant, you'll find you can eat well on the Whole Body Reset.

❏ We can eat real, normal, everyday foods: There are no special products or expensive supplements or exotic "superfoods"—just great, delicious food you'll find at your local supermarket and favorite restaurants. (Yes, even fast-food restaurants!)

❏ We can eat when we want: We don't have to fast or cleanse, or restrict ourselves to "on" or "off" hours or days. There aren't any tricky phases to navigate.

❏ This program is safe, healthy, and effective, and approved by top researchers in the fields of aging, nutrition, and weight management.

To prove just how effective this plan is, AARP solicited employees ages fifty to seventy-five to take part in the first national pilot of the Whole Body Reset. More than one hundred employees embarked on a twelve-week health journey designed to stop, and even reverse, age-related weight gain and muscle loss. Even as they ate and exercised to build and preserve muscle mass, participants reported an average weight loss of more than five pounds, with one in three losing ten pounds or more. In the coming pages, you'll meet some of these folks—people just like you and me—and discover how easy it was for them to tweak their diets and earn life-altering results.

The Whole Body Reset works. It worked for me. It worked for our exclusive AARP test panel.

And it can work for you.

P.S.: Take the action! During our hugely successful Whole Body Reset pilot, we sent our panelists weekly, two-minute exercises designed to help them turn the ideas in this program into simple but life-changing steps toward taking back control of their health. You'll find these "action steps" at the end of each of the first twelve chapters in the book. So grab a pencil and give them a try: They'll make your journey even easier!

Top Ten Benefits of the Whole Body Reset

1. Prevent and reverse age-related weight gain
2. Support and regulate the immune system
3. Curtail age-related muscle loss
4. Protect against loss of mobility
5. Bolster cognitive function
6. Promote bone health
7. Support robust cardiovascular health, including healthy blood pressure
8. Stabilize blood sugar
9. Improve general digestive health
10. Boost vitality, alertness, and engagement

— The Whole Body Reset at a Glance —

Number of meals: 3 (breakfast, lunch, and dinner)

At least 25 grams of protein at each meal for women, at least 30 grams for men. Each meal will include at least 5 grams of fiber. (Don't worry, this is easy!)

Number of snacks: 1–2

Each snack will give you an additional 7 or more grams of protein and 2 or more grams of fiber.

Foods to focus on:

❏ **Animal and plant proteins.** Lean meat, fish, poultry, eggs, nuts, and beans all figure in our daily protein strategy, although you can reach this goal even if you follow a strict vegetarian or vegan lifestyle (we'll show you how).

❏ **Dairy.** You'll gain additional benefits if a portion of your protein intake comes from dairy foods, which will give you crucial muscle-building, disease-fighting nutrients like calcium, vitamin D, and magnesium. Can't tolerate lactose? We've got you covered (see page 64).

❏ **High-fiber grains, cereals, beans, and nuts.** Potent fiber sources, these plant foods will keep your energy high and help support fat fighting, muscle maintenance, and gut health.

❏ **Colorful fruits and vegetables.** You need to eat more now that you're a little older. As we age, our ability to extract nutrients from food diminishes, so it's important to snack on lots of colorful plant foods throughout the day, giving you fiber as well as vital minerals, vitamins, and other nutrients.

❑ **Healthy fats and oils from omega-3-rich seafoods, nuts, olives, and avocado.** Two servings a day will help keep you lean and sharp.

❑ **Calorie-free drinks.** The Whole Body Reset promotes increased consumption of water, still and sparkling—try it with a slice of fruit!—as well as unsweetened tea and coffee.

Secret weapon: Protein breakfast smoothies. The easiest, most efficient way to make every day a muscle-building, fat-burning day.

Foods to avoid: Highly processed foods and calorie-laden drinks. (Don't worry—you won't feel deprived! You can still find plenty of ready-to-eat treats in your local market or online store. See Chapter 8 for the amazing Magic Supermarket Label Decoder.)

Exercise: Whatever fits your lifestyle and your body—walking, running, biking, hiking, dancing in the kitchen—along with some strength and resistance training. Shoot for about thirty minutes a day, about five days per week. (We make it easy to do and easy to fit into your day—see Chapter 12, Your Whole Body Fitness Plan.)

Phases, restrictions, specific meal timings, "superfoods," and gimmicks: None.

Chapter 1

The Age-Defying Magic of Protein Timing

The Shocking New Breakthrough in Nutrition

If you feel helpless and hopeless about your weight, you're not alone. In the United States, nearly 43 percent of adults aged forty to fifty-nine are overweight or obese. Among those sixty and older, 41 percent are obese. Among adult Hispanics and non-Hispanic Blacks, rates are even more dire, especially for women: 54 percent of adult Black women and 51 percent of adult Hispanic women are obese.

Chances are, you've already tried a bunch of other diets. And workouts. And superfoods. And even if you've lost weight successfully in the past, I can almost guarantee that you've since put those pounds—and more—back on your frame. In fact, one study[1] of more than 8,800 people found that those who had been on a diet in the previous year were significantly more likely to gain weight than those who had not. And the more diets you go on, the greater your likelihood of gaining weight in the future.

That's because traditional weight-loss diets trigger our bodies to grow fatter in three specific ways.

The first is that, by restricting calories, a traditional diet sends your body the message that it needs to be prepared to live through times of famine. Once your body receives that signal, it automatically turns down your resting metabolism—the number of calories your body burns while you're sleeping, sitting at the computer, or binge-watching TV shows. So as great as it might feel to lose a few pounds by cutting calories or skipping meals or restricting foods, what you've done in reality is to reduce the number of calories your body burns each and every day, setting you up for future weight gain.

"Once I knew what my go-to foods were, it was fairly simple. I've made permanent changes to what and how I eat."

—Tracy Eichelberger, age 55, Washington, DC
Dropped 9 pounds on the 12-week test panel

The second is that when we go on a diet, we don't just lose fat. Most of us lose muscle, too, and muscle is more metabolically active than fat. Once we're into our mid-forties or so, muscle loss is already an insidious problem we must battle against on a daily basis. Because muscle plays a huge role in preventing belly fat, the more muscle we lose, the more belly fat we'll gain in response.

The third and perhaps most important reason is that most diets are built for the general public, not for people in midlife. And our bodies at midlife ARE different.

But not in a bad way.

In fact, as we enter midlife, our bodies undergo an upgrade of sorts. They transition from old-school muscle cars—the type that run best on regular gas—to high-performance sports coupes. And high-performance vehicles require high-performance fuel.

Consider:

❑ As we get older, our body's ability to turn protein into muscle is reduced (a phenomenon known as "anabolic resistance"). This process starts as early as our thirties and accelerates with age. Our protein needs skyrocket, as our bodies are beset by age-related muscle loss. New research shows that people in their fifties, sixties, and seventies may need considerably more protein than those in their twenties and thirties—and far more than current RDA guidelines recommend.[2] And not just a steak at dinner; we need to spread protein throughout the day if we want to hold on to our life-giving muscle; science shows that those who retain muscle as they age lower their risk of obesity, heart disease, even dementia.

❑ As we pass midlife, our ability to extract nutrients from food diminishes, so "nutrient density"—the notion of making your calories count, nutrition-wise—becomes a critical issue. In particular, vitamin D, calcium, magnesium, and vitamin B12 often become more difficult for us to access—even if we're getting enough of them. And these nutrients are crucial to helping us hold on to muscle and prevent fat gain. That's another reason why we need more protein and dairy, as well as more fruits and vegetables. Indeed, researchers have recently discovered that the more fruits and vegetables older adults eat, the lower their degree of muscle loss as they age.[3]

❑ Americans eat only about 16 grams of fiber per day—not nearly enough to keep our weight steady. A lack of fiber may be one of the biggest reasons we can't drop pounds. One weight-loss study of individuals with metabolic syndrome (a combination of health factors including excess belly fat and high cholesterol, blood pressure, and blood sugar) found that eating 30 grams of

---

Why the Whole Body Reset? And Why Now?

We asked our panelists why they needed the Whole Body Reset. Here are some of their responses:

- "I'm getting married to my partner in July and am trying to lose about ten pounds before then."
- "It is simple: I want to see my grandchildren grow up!"
- "I'm planning a hiking vacation this summer and know by losing weight I'll have more endurance and enjoy myself much more."
- "As a type 2 diabetic, I am always looking for ways to control and reduce my A1C."
- "I have lost some weight but the last ten to fifteen pounds are so stubborn."

---

fiber per day, without dieting, was nearly as effective as following a diet that cut sugar, fat, salt, and alcohol. And yet—shockingly—the USDA guidelines actually recommend we reduce fiber intake as we age! No wonder we're gaining weight!

All these weight-related factors, and their effect on midlife Americans, have been extensively researched. They just haven't been widely reported on. Until now. And no diet takes these surprising and significant differences in our bodies into account. Until now.

The Unique Promise of the Whole Body Reset

Enter the Whole Body Reset, and the magic of protein timing. It's a very simple way of eating that helps your body resist age-related muscle loss—even while you're burning fat and losing weight. Protein timing isn't a new concept, and it isn't a gimmick. It's a long-proven approach to maintaining and even growing lean muscle tissue. Mostly, it's been used by young athletes to improve performance, including muscular endurance, strength, power, and cardiovascular health.

But more and more evidence is showing that as we get older, timing our protein intake is no longer just a matter of being able to jump higher or run longer. Because of the way our bodies change with age, protein timing becomes crucial to keeping us lean, healthy, and disease-free. Eating the right amount of protein at healthy intervals means significant weight loss with no rebound weight gain. One study even found that overweight adults 50+ became both leaner and physically stronger when they started using protein timing.[4]

Here's why: When you were in your twenties, you could turn a glass of milk into muscle. Just a single cup of milk—with its 8 grams of protein—could get your body's muscle-maintenance process revving. But by the time we reach our thirties or so, we've already begun to see that ability fade—the aforementioned anabolic resistance. Metaphorically speaking, that glass of milk no longer boots up your muscle-building operating system. You need a bigger dose. The "make muscle" button has to be pushed harder and harder as we get older in order to make the process turn on.

This is a huge issue, because our bodies are constantly breaking down and rebuilding muscle tissue. But if you're not able to convert the food you eat into new muscle, then you're tearing down faster than you're building back up.

And by the time we're in our fifties, the problem has gotten severe enough that many of us have already begun losing significant amounts of muscle mass—leading to weight gain and all sorts of bad health outcomes. (You'll read how this process increases our risk of heart disease, diabetes, and Alzheimer's, among many other issues, in the coming chapters.)

But we can stop this slow descent into muscle loss and weight gain. This process is reversible. And so easily!

All we need to do is to up our protein intake to 25 to 30 grams per meal, and our bodies respond the same way a younger person's would. Indeed, one study found that when people in their sixties combined a high-quality protein meal and resistance exercise, their bodies responded in the same way as the bodies of people in their twenties.[5]

Let's say that again: If you eat the right amount of quality protein, your body responds as if it were forty to fifty years younger. Voilà. The Whole Body Reset.

This isn't a controversial point or some sort of far-out idea, by the way. It's the official position of PROT-AGE, an association of gerontologists and nutritionists. It recently reaffirmed that older people should eat about 1 to 1.2 grams of protein per kilogram of body weight—or roughly 0.5 to 0.6 grams per pound. But they also concluded that 25 to 30 grams of protein per meal was crucial[6] for older people to reach their anabolic threshold—the point at which muscle can be maintained. And maintaining that muscle mass is what we're after.

And don't get the idea that this is some sort of "high-protein diet." The average person following this plan won't actually eat much, if any, more protein on a given day than he or she does already. But what will happen is that the timing and concentration of that protein is going to change. And the results will be extraordinary.

Nor is the Whole Body Reset one of those miserable "low-carb" or "low-fat" diets. No, there will be plenty of comforting carbs, including whole grain bread, with an emphasis on high-fiber cereals, beans and rice, and plenty of satisfying, healthy fats as well. And of course, delicious salads and flavorful fruits and vegetables. Once you understand the power of protein timing, you'll see how easy it is to build nutritious and satisfying meals around all your favorite foods. Nothing is—pardon the pun—off the table.*

Essentially, to stay lean and strong, our bodies need to be treated more like those of elite athletes. If you think of your midlife body in this way—as an upgraded model that needs special care, in the form of quality protein and higher-nutrient foods—you'll be amazed at how well it can perform and how good it can look. More important, you'll see many of the markers of age and ill health—blood pressure levels, cholesterol counts, blood sugar readings, and the like—come back under control. These numbers are the warning lights on your dashboard. They're not telling you that you're getting old. They're telling you that the very cool, upgraded vehicle currently transporting you around simply needs better care.

For people at midlife, protein timing begins at breakfast. Indeed, research shows that women who eat less than 25 grams of protein in the morning (for men, it's 30 grams) will probably be in muscle-loss mode all day.[7] So if your day typically starts with little more than a croissant and coffee, or even with a bowl of oatmeal and fruit, you'll find that single biggest step you can take on your midlife weight-loss journey will come on your very first meal of day one. Of course, your physical size and features need to be taken into account: If you're a ballerina or a linebacker, you may need a little less or a little more protein at each meal. But studies suggest that even healthy older adults suffer from an impaired response to protein intake below 20 grams when compared to their younger peers.[8]

To get your day started, we've got plenty of protein-powered

---

* Diets that are too high in protein may pose issues for people who have underlying kidney disease. As with any health and nutrition change, it is important to talk to your doctor about your protein needs and intake as you age.

> ## "I felt like I had more control over my eating and my physicality."
>
> **Beth Daniels, age 57, Silver Spring, Maryland**
> Dropped 19 pounds on the 12-week test panel
>
> "I had always been able to lose weight when I wanted to," says Beth. "Like a normal person, my weight would go up and down. But once I turned fifty, it changed." Suddenly she no longer had control over her weight, and she needed to make a change. She also wanted to be thinner at her wedding, which was just a few months away.
>
> The Whole Body Reset appealed to Beth for a number of reasons, but one of the most enticing was the recipes. "There are recipes I still make years later! They were extremely helpful because I need to be told how to cook stuff. It made me feel like I had more control over my eating habits and my physicality. And they were tasty!" Plus, she felt more comfortable eating out at restaurants, always knowing what she could order that would keep her body nourished. "You have some very good tips on eating at restaurants while staying on the plan."
>
> Within weeks, Beth noticed a change in how she felt. "I wasn't sluggish. My sleep was good and I had improvements in my mood. I just noticed that it was easier for me to move around—I felt lighter in my person. It was very motivating, and it just made me feel more engaged."
>
> But Beth was surprised to see that while she was changing on the outside, healthy changes were happening inside as well. "I was using my Fitbit and I realized my resting heart rate was noticeably lower. It was usually around seventy beats per minute, but it dropped down to about sixty-four."

breakfast ideas: easy-to-whip-up recipes and even some ideas on what you can order at your favorite chain restaurant.

Too busy to cook or even hit the drive-thru? To make muscle-up mornings even easier, we include nine breakfast protein smoothie recipes in Chapter 14. A smoothie for breakfast may be the fastest, easiest, and most delicious way to reset your whole body for muscle maintenance and weight control. Even if you don't eat dairy.

Let me say it again: That traditionally healthy breakfast, even if you're eating the high-fiber oat-bran cereal your cardiologist recommends, isn't, in fact, healthy enough.

Not for someone your age, or mine.

What to Expect on the Whole Body Reset

As you can already see, the Whole Body Reset is not a traditional diet plan.

It's not a diet you'll "go on," only to one day "go off." It won't cause you to yo-yo between weight loss and those inevitable rebound pounds. Instead, it's a sustainable, lifelong approach to eating designed to help you halt age-related weight gain in its tracks and then gently guide you to a lifelong path of slow and easy weight loss. The Whole Body Reset isn't about depriving you of foods; it's about increasing the number of healthy, life-sustaining foods you do eat. You can eat cake at the birthday party, and you don't have to hide under the couch when the pizza arrives. You just have to make sure to eat the nutrients you need each day to keep your body lean and strong.

Instead of sacrifice and restriction, the Whole Body Reset simply asks us to eat plenty of healthy, satisfying protein, timed throughout the day. You can put an emphasis on dairy—milk, cheese, and yogurt—as well as meat, fish, and poultry, if those foods fit your body and lifestyle. Or use the many plant-based suggestions in this program to create a vegetarian- or even vegan-friendly version. (You'll find both dairy-based and vegan protein smoothie recipes starting on page 243.)

Quality protein. Fiber. Healthy fats. Vitamins and minerals, particularly potassium, magnesium, folate, vitamin D, and calcium. These and other essential life-giving substances are packed into the Whole Body Reset in ways that make them easy for our bodies to access, digest, and put to use. As we get older, we have difficulty absorbing and using many of these nutrients, so to stay lean, fit, and healthy, people our age simply need more of them than younger folks do.

We'll eat three satisfying meals and at least one belly-filling snack each day, packing in the nutrients our bodies need in a way that eliminates cravings, hunger pangs, and any sense of deprivation.

As our pilot study proved, we can stay full and satisfied even as the weight falls off as if by magic. Within the first two weeks, belly fat will begin to disappear. We'll feel less bloated. We'll wake up each day looking forward to seeing how much stronger and healthier we feel.

Even as these clear differences in our appearance are happening, our bodies can change dramatically on the inside as well. Blood glucose levels may drop. Cholesterol levels may drop. On a cellular level, we may develop healthier, more numerous, more vibrant mitochondria—the microscopic engines of energy and youth.[9]

Muscle tissue, which has been deteriorating since our thirties, will begin to grow stronger as we improve our protein intake and combine it with a simple exercise plan.

And it will happen not because we are denying ourselves certain foods or because we're trying to eat less. Just the opposite. It will happen because we're finally feeding our bodies more of the nutrients that our modern food culture, and even the recommendations of our government, has been depriving us of.

The only thing you really need to do on the Whole Body Reset is to make sure you hit your protein and fiber numbers while eating more good, healthy food. And the secret behind this program is to identify the premium nutrients your premium body needs more of, and find simple, clever, and delicious ways to fit more of them into your day.

So get ready for a weight-loss revolution. The Whole Body Reset is here.

— ACTION STEP # 1 —

Eating 25 to 30 grams of protein at each meal, especially at breakfast, is critical as we get older. To begin focusing on this goal, take a moment to list three ways you can get 25 to 30 grams of protein at each meal. To plan out your proteins, refer to our Complete Whole Body Reset Mix 'N' Match Meal Maker on page 341. (Don't forget that protein comes from various sources—not just meat, fish, and dairy but whole grains, beans, and nuts as well.) Or steal any of the recipes from Chapter 14!

Breakfast

1. _____

2. _____

3. _____

Lunch

1. _____

2. _____

3. _____

Dinner

1. _____

2. _____

3. _____

The Story of Two "Healthy" Diets

Meet Joan, age fifty-six.

Joan lives what she believes is a pretty healthy lifestyle. She runs a few times a week, rides her bike, and walks whenever she can, and she tries to eat healthfully. In fact, by most standards, Joan's diet is top-notch.

But . . . Joan has gained weight since she hit her late forties—not a lot, but a pound or two every year. Today she's fifteen pounds heavier than she was on her forty-fifth birthday, and she can't figure out why. She eats the same as she always has. She exercises the same. But she keeps gaining weight.

What's going on?

Joan's next-door neighbor, Maria, is the same age. But unlike Joan, her weight is stable; in fact, she's still fitting into the jeans she wore a decade earlier. She spends about the same amount of time exercising as Joan does, but while she also bikes and walks a lot, Maria is not a runner. Instead, she does resistance training in the form of yoga and Pilates.

Joan and Maria eat very similar diets, and they have similar fitness schedules. But there are subtle differences. And those differences help to explain why Joan keeps gaining weight around her midsection, and Maria doesn't. Can you see why?

Joan's Breakfast:
Oatmeal cooked in water (½ cup uncooked), with ¼ cup blueberries and ½ cup skim milk
9 g protein, 5 g fiber, 205 calories

Joan's breakfast is the spitting image of "healthy," at least according to most nutrition experts. And she's getting enough cholesterol-lowering fiber to make her cardiologist happy. But she's starting her day with less than 10 grams of protein. That means that today is going to be a muscle-loss day for our friend Joan, no matter what else happens for the next twenty-four hours.

Maria's Breakfast:
Orange Crush Smoothie (recipe, page 248)
36 g protein, 8 g fiber, 422 calories

A protein smoothie is just about the fastest, easiest way to start your day in muscle-maintenance mode. This smoothie combines Greek yogurt and vanilla whey protein powder (both great sources of calcium as well) with a splash of orange juice, peaches, banana, and ground flax seeds for a powerful fiber boost. If Maria keeps up her protein intake throughout the day and does some moderate exercise, today is going to be a muscle-positive day. Plus, Maria is weighting her calories toward the morning, which will help keep hunger at bay later on.

Joan's Snack:
Granola bar and a bunch of grapes
2 g protein, 2 g fiber, 146 calories

Granola bars are a "health halo" food. They sound healthy, but that's only if you're comparing them to Snickers bars. And while grapes are good for you, they're among the lowest-fiber fruits.

Maria's Snack:
½ cup 2% cottage cheese with 1 cup strawberries and ¼ cup mixed nuts
18 g protein, 3 g fiber, 307 calories

Dairy always makes for a great snack choice, because it guarantees a protein punch and delivers bone-preserving calcium and magnesium. Maria pairs it with nuts and berries for fiber.

Joan's Lunch:
1 cup green salad (lettuce, shredded carrot, and sliced
cucumber) with ¼ cup chickpeas, 1 oz cheddar cheese, and
1 tbsp low-fat Italian dressing
1 cup tomato basil soup with 6 wheat crackers
13 g protein, 4 g fiber, 361 calories

Oh, how Joan used to love grabbing a burger at lunchtime with the gang. But with her weight becoming more and more of an issue (did we mention her cholesterol, blood pressure, and blood sugar levels are all higher than a decade ago?), she's a martyr to low-cal eating. Poor Joan!

Maria's Lunch:
Wendy's Chili (small) plus a half order of Southwest Avocado
Chicken Salad
33 g protein, 6 g fiber, 425 calories

While Joan's eating a sad soup and salad at her desk, Maria's grabbing a quick lunch with colleagues at a local fast-food joint. She's getting her protein and fiber from both the chili and the side salad, plus plenty of nutritional power from the beans, avocado, and other vegetables. That doesn't seem fair, does it?

Joan's Afternoon Pick-Me-Up:
Vanilla latte, medium, with 2% milk
3 g protein, 0 g fiber, 350 calories

Eating a "healthy," low-cal diet means Joan often feels low on energy. A delicious, blended coffee drink gives her the shot of energy she needs. But while she's getting some protein from the milk, this coffee drink, with its four pumps of vanilla syrup, is a big gulp of calories with no fiber.

Maria's Afternoon Pick-Me-Up:
Cup of green tea
0 g protein, 0 g fiber, 0 calories

Thanks to the protein and fiber Maria's had, she doesn't feel the need to snack after lunch. A calorie-free drink also helps Maria stay hydrated—something that can be more difficult for us as we get older.

Joan's Dinner:
Turkey burger on a hamburger bun topped with a slice of tomato, lettuce, and 1 oz cheddar cheese with a side of 1 cup of steamed broccoli
36 g protein, 5 g fiber, 463 calories

Like most Americans, Joan eats the majority of her protein at dinner. But it's not enough to make up for the protein she lacked earlier in the day. And while a side of veggies is great, she needs to look for more opportunities to slide hunger-squelching, gut-healthy fiber into her day.

Maria's Dinner:
Turkey burger on a hamburger bun topped with a slice of tomato, lettuce, 2 tbsp guacamole, and 1 oz part-skim mozzarella cheese, with a side of 1 cup of steamed broccoli
37 g protein, 7 g fiber, 478 calories

Just 2 tablespoons of an avocado gives you 2 grams of fiber. This simple tweak helps Maria keep her hunger under control for the rest of the evening, while Joan goes to bed dreaming of an ice-cream sundae.

Joan's Daily Total:
63 grams protein
16 grams fiber
1,525 calories

Maria's Daily Total:
124 grams protein
24 grams fiber
1,632 calories

Of course, Joan won't have that sundae, because she's watching her weight. But she's not eating enough protein to keep her from losing valuable lean-muscle tissue, nor enough fiber to fight chronic inflammation, a condition that helps add to muscle loss and fat gain. Plus, no matter how many miles Joan walks, runs or bikes, she's not engaging in resistance exercises that help keep her muscles strong.

The result: Tomorrow, while Maria wakes up ready for another day of muscle maintenance and weight control, Joan will wake up with just a tiny bit less muscle, and a tiny bit more fat, than she did the day before. Even though Maria ate slightly more calories than Joan, it's Maria who is on the glidepath to long-term health and weight control.

Source for nutrients: ESHA Research (ESHA.com). Nutrients can vary depending on brand, size, and ingredients. Check packaging for exact amounts.

Chapter 2

Our Changing Bodies, Our Changing Needs

Why We Need to Eat Differently Today than We Did in Our Thirties

Consider the egg.

You might call it nature's perfect food, a staple of diets up and down the food chain, for species as diverse as ants, fish, snakes, ravens, racoons, polar bears, and the average Joe idling in the drive-thru at your local McDonald's. One nice, big chicken egg packs 6 grams of protein, as well as other vital nutrients like calcium, vitamin D, and choline.

But if eggs are a near-universal food, what happens to our bodies when we eat one can vary wildly, depending on which side of age fifty we happen to fall. So consider your next egg in a slightly different light: a scrambled, hard-boiled, easy-over metaphor for how your body ages, and why the information in this book is so critical to your future health and your battle against weight gain.

Let's say you and your child meet up for breakfast. Let's call him Dom: He's twenty-five, a hard worker, a dedicated son, and you're proud of him. You're not loving his current girlfriend, and you wish he'd spend less time nurturing his beard, but beyond that he's pretty great. You see reflections of you and your spouse in his eyes, and every time he smiles, he fills you with joy. And, like you, he loves his eggs sunny-side up. You both order a couple, with a slice of whole wheat toast and a cup of coffee, and talk about the events of the day. After you eat, you chat for a while about the extended family, the weather, the local gossip. Then you pick up the tab (of course) and the two of you walk to your cars, linger in the sunshine for ten minutes, hug goodbye, and go your separate ways.

You enjoyed the same start to the day, savored the same breakfast and the same beautiful morning sun. But in the coming hours, your bodies are going to respond to this morning very differently.

Once you understand those differences, you'll instantly understand how to adjust your diet to your changing body's needs. It's not rocket science. But just a few simple tweaks to your diet can give you a Whole Body Reset.

Calorie Burn Conundrum

For breakfast, you and your son both ate about 270 calories—about 140 from the two eggs, a little less than 70 from the slice of toast, and perhaps another 60 calories from two teaspoons of butter used to fry up the eggs and slather your toast.

When those calories hit your son's body, they land like snowflakes on a hot car hood. Your engine, however, doesn't run as hot, for a number of reasons.

Certainly, we tend to be less active as we age. The responsibilities of work and parenthood that set in for most of us play a role, slowing us down as we approach middle age and keeping us sedentary as we get older. And as we age, the aches and pains of old injuries, the appearance of new health issues, and our increasing girth can make it harder to be as physically engaged as we once were.

But physical activity makes up a minority of our daily calorie burn. Between 60 and 80 percent of the calories we burn each day come from the simple business of staying alive: keeping our hearts beating, our lungs pumping, our organs squirting out hormones. Regenerating cells, sending electrical impulses throughout the body, even growing our fingernails—all that miraculous stuff takes a lot of energy. This is known as the resting metabolic rate (RMR).

Until very recently, it was believed that RMR slowed automatically during middle age, but a shocking study published in the journal *Science* in August 2021 ("Daily Energy Expenditure Through the Human Life Course") called that assumption into question. Looking at data from more than 6,400 individuals across twenty-nine countries, researchers found that our individual cells rev at pretty much the same rate in our forties and fifties as they did in our twenties—indeed, our metabolic rate doesn't start to drop off until about age sixty or so, when it begins to drop at a rate of .07 percent a year, indefinitely.

The study's lead researcher, Herman Pontzer, associate professor of evolutionary anthropology and global health at Duke University, was as surprised by the results as anyone. "I'm in my forties so I expected to see some evidence to back up my subjective experience that my metabolism is slowing down. It feels that way to me!" he told AARP. "But it's not really what's happening."

So what is happening?

"Your stress level, your schedule, your hormone levels, your energy levels are different in your forties or fifties compared to your twenties," says Pontzer, who is also the author of *Burn: New Research Blows the Lid Off How We Really Burn Calories, Lose Weight, and Stay Healthy*. These factors can lead us to burn slightly fewer calories each day, while hormonal changes may make it harder for us to balance our energy intake. Testosterone levels, for example, are highest in our twenties, then decline with age. Testosterone is one factor that determines how many of the calories we consume end up as lean muscle tissue, and how many end up as belly fat.

So the growing girth you notice—the difference between your body now and your body when you were Dom's age—isn't due to metabolism. Something else is at play.

Something you can actually control.

Let's dive a little deeper.

Different Ages, Different Muscles

Within an hour of eating breakfast, your twentysomething child's body will have reached peak concentrations of amino acids[1]—the components of protein that are the building blocks of muscle.

In fact, you could call protein the building blocks of your whole body, since it's also vital to dozens of tasks related to youth, vibrancy, and overall health: maintaining bone density, regulating blood sugar and hormone production, repairing damaged tissue, manufacturing collagen, supporting the immune system, keeping hair and nails strong, and more.

And Dom's body utilizes the protein from breakfast—12 or so grams from the eggs and 4.5 grams from the whole wheat toast—with maximum efficiency. Dom digests the protein into amino acids, which are transported throughout his body via the circulatory system and then reconfigured to form healthy new muscle cells. This whole process is known as "protein synthesis."[2]

But as we discussed in Chapter 1, while this life-sustaining process is going on inside Dom's body, it actually hasn't kicked into gear inside yours.

As we noted, the human body is constantly breaking down and building up muscle. But when the destruction of muscle outstrips its rate of repair over the long term, that eventually leads to a loss of muscle tissue. The scientific term for this gradual loss of muscle over the years is *sarcopenia*. For those of us at midlife and beyond, this age-related process is reshaping our bodies every day. An easy place to spot its effects is in the shoulders of older people—once broad and strong, shoulders can narrow with time, because the muscular scaffolding needed to keep the shoulders big and strong is weakened and diminished. Research findings vary, but at some point between age thirty and forty, adults begin to lose 3 to 8 percent of their muscle mass each decade. Sarcopenia is when this process kicks into overdrive: 72 percent of men and 44 percent of women over age sixty-five can be characterized as at least moderately sarcopenic, according to one study.[3] That's what the Whole Body Reset protects you from—sarcopenia and its even more evil twin, dynapenia.

While sarcopenia is the loss of muscle mass and function, dynapenia is the loss of muscle strength.[4] It moves on us even more quickly; in their legs alone, older adults lose muscular strength two to five times faster than they lose muscle mass, according to a study in the *American Journal of Clinical Nutrition*.[5] And the effects can be devastating; we may begin struggling with the daily tasks of life, not to mention the fun stuff we want to keep doing, from hiking to biking to chasing grandkids around the yard. Research shows that about one in six women and up to one in ten men aged sixty-five or older cannot kneel or stoop down or lift a mere ten pounds. This is the first step toward frailty, a weakened and delicate condition none of us wants to find ourselves in; it puts us at increased risk of injury, disability, and even death.

The loss of strength is caused in part by our aging nervous system. The "wires" that send signals throughout our bodies may not be able to transmit those signals as efficiently as they once did. Power is generated by speed. In our youth, we said "jump!" and our muscles asked "how high!" As we get older, we say "jump!" and our muscles say, "er, what?"

When your muscles wither, so do your opportunities to enjoy the world around you. Muscles are essential to keeping you upright and moving, independent and in control, for decades to come. And it's not exaggerating to say they can save your life. In one study, men with the most muscle mass at age forty-five had an 81 percent lower risk of heart disease than those with the least muscle mass.[6] Muscle loss also puts us at risk of weight gain and even diabetes, because low muscle mass increases our risk of insulin resistance, which translates to increased glucose levels. Age-related muscle loss can also make you feel tired, cause balance problems, and increase the risk of falls. A lack of muscle puts you at greater risk for osteoporosis and life-altering disability. It has even been associated with an increase in your risk of dementia.[7]

For all those reasons and more, it's no wonder low muscle strength is associated with an elevated risk of death, regardless of general health levels, according to a study of 4,449 people ages fifty and older.[8] Even cardio exercise, important for heart health as well as balance, doesn't appear to protect you if you allow your strength levels to deteriorate. And a predominant reason for that loss of muscle size, strength, and function has to do with our diminished ability to process protein. It's this aspect of aging that the Whole Body Reset is designed to counteract.

Of course, a lot of different factors go into determining how quickly we gain weight as we age. But the physiological changes described above illustrate exactly why we need to treat our older bodies as high-performance vehicles. We need greater amounts of nutrition for fewer calories, and we need to time our meals so we're always in muscle-building mode.

Fortunately, eating to preserve lean muscle and melt away fat doesn't require us to focus on exotic superfoods or weird ingredients. Just turn to page 36 to find the Quick Whole Body Reset Mix 'N' Match Meal Maker. It's an at-a-glance guide to fueling your body properly, every time. Find the Complete Mix 'N' Match Meal Maker in Appendix 1.

If you've got a favorite food, it's probably in the Meal Maker.

— ACTION STEP #2 —

The easiest way to add more nutrients into your day is to eat fewer processed foods (the stuff with lots of ingredients and empty calories) and more whole foods (the stuff with just one ingredient). Let's discover how easy this can be.

Name three processed foods you can find in your pantry right now, and name three whole-food options (or combinations of whole foods) you could substitute for them. For example: Swap energy bars for a mix of nuts and berries; exchange fruit spreads for real fruits; toss out flavored oatmeal or yogurt for plain, topped with fruit and nuts and a sprinkle of cinnamon; or dump the premade salad dressing for olive oil and vinegar.

	Processed Food		**Whole Food**
Swap	_____	for	_____
Swap	_____	for	_____
Swap	_____	for	_____

The Quick Whole Body Reset Mix 'N' Match Meal Maker

We're blessed to live in a time when nearly every kind of comestible known to humans is a mere click or two away, and many neighborhoods offer both supermarkets and big-box stores that present a glorious cornucopia of foodstuffs. There's so much good, nutritious stuff to eat—you just need to put it in smart, healthy combinations that you eat throughout the day, giving your body the nutrients it needs without adding empty calories. Note: This is just a partial list of the possibilities. A complete list of proteins, fiber—vegetables, fruits, and starches—and fats appears on page 341.

Two Easy Steps

1. Start with protein—25 to 30 grams at each meal, with two to three servings of dairy a day. A 4-ounce serving of meat or fish delivers 14 to 25 grams.

2. Aim for at least 5 grams of fiber at each meal from veggies, fruits, and starches. Choose veggies of various colors to fill half your plate. Pick two to four fruits a day. Add whole grains to fill out your meals.

Deck of Cards

A simple way to eyeball protein is that a cooked portion of red meat or poultry should be a little bigger than the size of a deck of playing cards, while a portion of fish is about the size of a checkbook.

Protein

Try to eat two to three servings of dairy a day, and two to three servings of omega-3-rich foods a week (salmon, tuna, mackerel, sardines, walnuts, or tofu): 25–30 grams of protein per meal, 7 grams per snack.

PROTEIN SOURCE	SERVING SIZE	PROTEIN (GRAMS)
Beans, black (cooked or canned)	½ cup	8
Beef, ground (85% lean)	4 oz	21
Beef jerky	1 oz	11
Chicken breast	3 oz	24
Egg	1	6
Milk	1 cup	8
Nut butter (almond, peanut)	2 tbsp	6–8
Nuts	1 oz	4–7
Salmon (cooked)	3 oz	23
Steak (filet, porterhouse, sirloin, strip, T-bone)	4 oz	25
Tempeh	3 oz	16
Tofu, firm	6 oz	17
Tuna, chunk light in water	3 oz	14
Turkey breast	3 oz	16
Turkey burger	3-oz patty	16
Yogurt, Greek, plain	1 cup	22

Fiber

Try to eat two to four servings of fruit and 1½ to 2½ cups of vegetables each day: at least 5 grams of fiber at each meal from a mix of veggies, fruits, and starches, 2 grams of fiber per snack.

VEGETABLE	SERVING SIZE	FIBER CONTENT (GRAMS)
Artichoke	1	7
Broccoli	1 cup, raw	3
Brussels sprouts	1 cup raw	3
Carrots	1 medium, or 7 baby carrots	2
Cauliflower	1 cup raw	2
Celery	3 stalks	2
Kale	1 cup raw	1
Peas	½ cup cooked	4
Peppers (red, orange, yellow)	1 cup raw	3
Winter squash (acorn, butternut)	1 cup raw	3

FRUIT	SERVING SIZE	FIBER CONTENT (GRAMS)
Apple	1 medium	5
Banana	1 medium	3
Blackberries	1 cup	4
Blueberries	1 cup	4
Cherries	12	2
Grapefruit	½	3
Orange	1	4
Strawberries	1 cup sliced	3

FIBER-RICH STARCH	SERVING SIZE	FIBER CONTENT (GRAMS)
Brown rice	⅓ cup cooked	1
Cereal, breakfast whole grain	1 cup	Varies by brand
Corn	½ cup	2
Corn tortilla (6 inch)	1	1
Crackers, multigrain	2	Varies by brand
Popcorn	2½ cups air-popped	3
Potato, sweet or white	½ potato	2–3
Whole wheat bread	1 slice	2–3
Whole wheat pasta	1 oz dry, ½ cup cooked	2

Chapter 3

Let's Spend a Day on the Whole Body Reset!

The How and Why of This Simple Meal Plan

Okay folks, pencils down!

Close that calorie-tracking app, put away that food journal. If your idea of "dieting" is to count calories, it's time to discover a different way of eating. It's time to stop focusing on eating "less" and start focusing on eating "more." More protein (especially at breakfast), more dairy, more colorful produce, more whole grains, more healthy fats, and wash it all down with more water.

Your upgraded, prime-time body needs more of all of these. That is how you will help preserve muscle, halt age-related weight gain, and enjoy lifelong health.

That said, it is necessary to eat fewer calories than you are expending if weight loss is a goal. But as you follow the Whole Body Reset, you will find that empty calories are naturally pushed out of your daily diet. As you reach your protein and fiber goals and stay hydrated throughout the day, you'll experience a decrease in hunger; as you focus on the foods you need, you'll lose the desire for the foods you don't need.

To make it simple, you can pick and choose options from the Complete Whole Body Reset Mix 'N' Match Meal Maker charts on page 341.

In an average day, a woman fifty or older following the Whole Body Reset plan will eat 75 to 100 grams of protein, spread throughout the day, and 20 to 25 grams of fiber, consuming about 1,600 calories a day, down from the average 2,200 calories that American women typically consume daily.

Men following the Whole Body Reset will eat 90 to 120 grams of protein, spread throughout the day, and 30 grams of fiber, consuming about 2,100 calories, down from an average of 2,400 for the typical American man.

So what will your meals look like in a typical day? There are a lot of simple and delicious ways to enjoy the Whole Body Reset. Here's a sample.

Breakfast

Women: at least 25 grams of protein and 5 grams of fiber, 350–450 calories*

Omelet with two eggs, 1 ounce low-fat mozzarella, 1 tablespoon chopped tomato, 5 sliced mushrooms

1 slice whole grain bread with 2 tablespoons avocado

Plus, 1 orange

Men: at least 30 grams of protein and 5 grams of fiber, about 500–550 calories*

Omelet with two eggs, 1 ounce low-fat mozzarella, 1 tablespoon chopped tomato, 5 sliced mushrooms

---

* Calorie estimates for each meal are general suggestions, not rules. Sometimes you'll eat more than this number of calories at a sitting, and sometimes less. That's okay: Focus on getting enough protein and fiber, including nutrient-rich produce, into your meals. The calories will take care of themselves.

2 slices whole grain bread with 4 tablespoons avocado

Plus, 1 orange

It seems that every day there's a new headline telling us that skipping breakfast will help us lose weight.

Breakfast used to have an unassailable rep as the most important meal of the day. Then, somewhere along the line, we started to hear differently.

Like about "intermittent fasting," a trendy way of eating in which you cut calories by restricting the times of day you're allowed to eat. Or fasting on certain days of the week and eating on others.

Well, while there's a lot of evidence that fasting has considerable health benefits for yeast, worms, fruit flies, and rodents, the National Institute on Aging says there's "no firm conclusion" on its effects on human health.

What we do know, however, is that not having protein for breakfast means you're setting yourself up for a day of muscle loss—and less muscle means more fat. Plus, eating breakfast is one of the best ways to ensure that you're getting the nutrients your body needs; one recent study found that those who skip meals early in the day generally get fewer nutrients and a lower-quality diet than those who skip meals later on.[1] Another study found that we actually burn more calories digesting breakfast than we do other meals.[2]

So there is no controversy, at least among the researchers who study age-related muscle loss: If you want to stay strong and active for years to come, eat a high-protein, fiber-packed breakfast every day.

I hear you night owls grumbling out there. You're not a morning person? Eating a big breakfast isn't your thing? You need more evidence? Okay: In one study, researchers put two sets of overweight or obese women (average age: forty-six) on exactly the same diet—1,400 calories a day for twelve weeks. Both sets ate 500-calorie lunches. One group ate 200 calories before lunch and 700 calories for dinner, while the other group ate 700 calories in the morning and 200 calories for dinner. At the end of twelve weeks, the big-breakfast group lost two and a half times more weight than the big-dinner group and more than three additional inches off their waists.[3]

Still, unless we spent the previous day chopping wood, 700 calories is a huge breakfast. As a solution, we've broken the morning meal into a breakfast and a snack. By filling the morning with high-protein, high-fiber food, we short-circuit binge eating later in the day and set ourselves up for the best possible results.

Snack

Women and men: at least 7 grams of protein and 2 grams of fiber, 250–300 calories

One 7-ounce container plain 2% yogurt

½ ounce chia seeds

1 tablespoon blueberries

The peak time for workplace snacking is 2 to 4 p.m., according to researchers. To break that habit, the Whole Body Reset places its emphasis on morning snacks, so our calorie intake begins to wind down after lunchtime. But don't feel locked into this timing; adjust your snack schedule to suit your lifestyle. What you snack on, not just when you snack, will also make a big difference in your appetite, satiation, satisfaction, and health. (You'll find a few quick snack ideas on page 46, and more elaborate suggestions in Chapter 14: Whole Body Recipes.)

Lunch

Women: at least 25 grams of protein and 5 grams of fiber, about 450–550 calories

Burrito bowl with chicken or vegetarian protein, cheese, guacamole, black beans, salsa, romaine lettuce, corn, and corn chips

Men: at least 30 grams of protein and 5 grams of fiber, about 550 calories

Burrito bowl with chicken or vegetarian protein, cheese, guacamole, black beans, salsa, romaine lettuce, corn, and corn chips

Midday is when most of us make our biggest nutritional mistakes. We're less than halfway through our day, we're too busy or too bored, we're distracted, and we just want the comfort of a delicious lunch to

Let Them Eat Cake

By eating the Whole Body Reset way, you've eliminated a lot of added sugar from your diet. So go ahead and enjoy a modest dessert if you want to at the end of the day. The key is to keep it small, and to sneak in nutrition wherever possible. Get a small ice cream or frozen yogurt (calcium!) and sprinkle some chopped peanuts (monounsaturated fats and protein!) and berries (fiber and phytonutrients!) on top.

If you love chocolate, look for high-quality dark chocolate that's at least 70 percent cacao. (Many quality chocolate makers now put the percentage of cacao—the bean from which chocolate is made—on the label. The greater the percentage of cacao, the greater the nutrition value.) A really high-quality dark chocolate can actually have health benefits, because it's low in sugar and packed with fiber and plant nutrients that have been shown to improve the health of blood vessels, reduce diabetes risk, protect nerves from inflammation, and possibly even protect against dementia.

take the edge off our day. If we're not home, often the choices available are questionable at best. But you can still enjoy lunch out with friends or co-workers by finding one of dozens of reasonable choices at popular restaurant chains (see Chapter 9) and convenience stores, as long as you remember to place an emphasis on getting the protein, fiber, and other nutrients that really matter.

Dinner

Women and men: at least 25 grams of protein for women and 30 for men, and 5 grams of fiber, about 400–500 calories

4 ounce grilled salmon

Roasted potatoes

Asparagus sautéed in 1 tablespoon olive oil with garlic

Optional dessert (not included in calorie count): ½ cup ice cream or 2 ounces of dark chocolate

---

Easy Snacks for Busy People

Each of these snacks provides at least 7 grams of protein, at least 2 grams of fiber, and between 210 and 300 calories.

- Trail mix of 2 tablespoons tart cherries, 2 tablespoons cashews, 20 pistachios, and ¼ cup wheat squares cereal
- ½ cup Greek yogurt with 1 cup blackberries and ¼ cup almonds
- 1 medium apple with 1 ounce cheddar cheese
- 1 medium banana with 2 tablespoons peanut butter
- 2 medium celery stalks, 2 tablespoons almond butter, 1 small apple
- ⅓ cup hummus with sliced carrot, cucumber, and red bell pepper

Dinner is where the majority of us currently eat more than half our protein. But we fall down in the vegetable department; the most commonly eaten vegetable in America is some form of fried potatoes. This ought to put you off your tots: A study of 4,440 people ages forty-five to seventy-nine found that, over an eight-year period, those who ate fried potatoes two or more times a week were twice as likely to die over the course of the study as those who ate less. Make French fries an occasional indulgence, and focus on getting greens and other colors onto your dinner plate.

To show how easy and delicious the Whole Body Reset can be, we've created our own chart to help you visualize the vast array of foods you can eat:

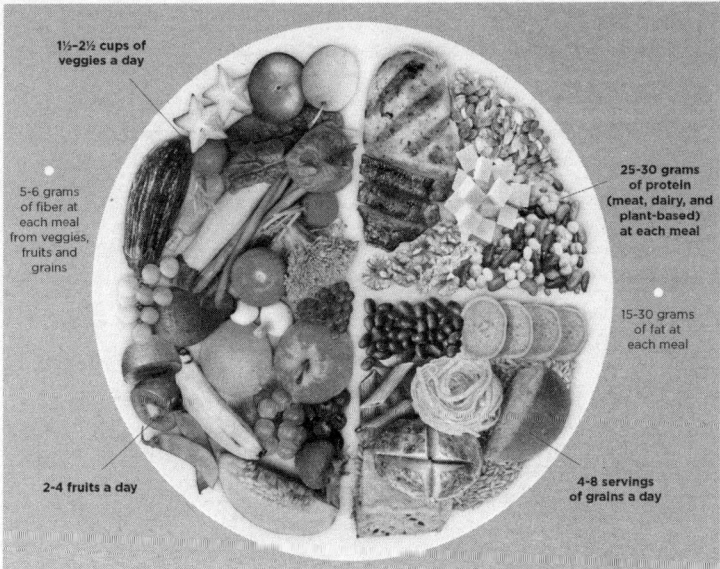

- 1½–2½ cups of veggies a day
- 5-6 grams of fiber at each meal from veggies, fruits and grains
- 2-4 fruits a day
- 25-30 grams of protein (meat, dairy, and plant-based) at each meal
- 15-30 grams of fat at each meal
- 4-8 servings of grains a day

— ACTION STEP #3 —

The Whole Body Reset isn't about subtracting, it's about adding. In many cases, we can reach optimum eating just by adding a little more protein and a little more fiber to each meal.

Think back on the last three meals you ate. Did each one reach at least 25 to 30 grams of protein and 5 grams of fiber? If not, what could you add to each to give it the boost it needs?

Your meal	Protein boost	Fiber boost
1. _____	_____	_____
_____	_____	_____
_____	_____	_____
2. _____	_____	_____
_____	_____	_____
_____	_____	_____
3. _____	_____	_____
_____	_____	_____
_____	_____	_____

A 7-Day Whole Body Reset Sample Menu

To show how simple, and how varied, the Whole Body Reset can be, we've created an easy seven-day sample menu. (And you'll find even more samples in Appendix 2!) You can follow this to the letter, or ignore it entirely and build your own fare from the Mix 'N' Match Meal Maker in Appendix 1. Just remember the simple tenets of the program:

Meals: Aim for at least 25 grams of protein for women, 30 for men, and at least 5 grams of fiber.

Snacks: Aim for at least 7 grams of protein and at least 2 grams of fiber.

SUNDAY

Breakfast
Protein-Punch Pancakes (recipe, page 256)
31 g protein, 8 g fiber, 434 calories

Snack
1 cup 2% milk with ⅓ bar 85% cacao dark chocolate
11 g protein, 4 g fiber, 312 calories

Lunch
Let's go watch the game at . . .
Buffalo Wild Wings: Six-Count Traditional Wings with Signature Sauce + Carrots and Celery with Fat-Free Ranch
32 g protein, 5 g fiber, 515 calories

Dinner
"I Ain't Cookin' Tonight" Taco Bowl with Pumpkin Seed Guac (recipes, pages 272 and 273)
27 g protein, 20 g fiber, 719 calories

MONDAY

Hey, why not try a "Meatless Monday"? Look how easy it is . . .

Breakfast
Muscled-Up Oats with Blueberries, Almonds, and Hemp Seeds (recipe, page 240)
28 g protein, 9 g fiber, 425 calories

Snack
Tart Cherry Trail Mix: Place 2 tablespoons dried sweetened tart cherries, 2 tablespoons cashews, 20 pistachios, and ¼ cup Wheat Chex cereal into a plastic bag, and shake until all ingredients are mixed.
7 g protein, 4 g fiber, 284 calories

Lunch
Let's stop off at Chipotle for a . . .
Sofritas Burrito Bowl with light cilantro-lime brown rice, black beans, fajita vegetables, fresh tomato salsa, Monterey Jack cheese
And add a clementine for even more nutrients: *1 g protein, 2 g fiber, 45 calories*
27 g protein, 14 g fiber, 645 calories

Dinner
Stone-Cold Soba Noodles (recipe, page 293)
25 g protein, 6 g fiber, 456 calories

TUESDAY

Breakfast
Kale and Hearty Smoothie (recipe, page 244)
25 g protein, 7 g fiber, 374 calories

Snack
6 whole grain crackers* with 1 oz thinly sliced Swiss cheese
11 g protein, 3 g fiber, 232 calories

* Nutrients were calculated for Triscuit crackers. Look for a cracker with at least 2 grams of fiber per serving, such as Wasa Light Rye and Mary's Gone Crackers.

Lunch
Salmon-I-Am Salad (recipe, page 283)
39 g protein, 6 g fiber, 390 calories

Dinner
Let's grab a fast dinner at . . .
Boston Market: Turkey Breast (regular) + Bacon Brussels Sprouts + Cornbread
39 g protein, 7 g fiber, 560 calories

WEDNESDAY

Breakfast
Three-egg omelet with 1 oz feta cheese, about 3 tablespoons avocado, and ¼ cup spinach
1¼ cups strawberries
25 g protein, 6 g fiber, 394 calories

Snack
½ cup plain Greek yogurt with 1 cup blackberries and ¼ cup almonds
18 g protein, 10 g fiber, 278 calories

Lunch
Doh! Forgot to pack lunch! Let's grab something quick at . . .
Subway: 6-inch Roast Beef Sub on 9-grain wheat bread with lettuce, tomatoes, green peppers, and cucumbers
Plus, an apple
26 g protein, 10 g fiber, 394 calories

Dinner
So Farro, So Good Chicken with Bok Choy (recipe, page 291)
36 g protein, 5 g fiber, 309 calories

THURSDAY

Breakfast
Crazy morning! Let's pick up breakfast at . . .
Dunkin': Kosher Southwest Veggie Power Breakfast Sandwich
25 g protein, 5 g fiber, 420 calories

Snack
1 apple with 2 tablespoons peanut butter
7 g protein, 7 g fiber, 270 calories

Lunch
**3½ ounces tuna, chunk light, in water with 1 tablespoon mayo
on 2 slices whole wheat toast**
Plus, a peach
35 g protein, 8 g fiber, 412 calories
Add 3 ounces baby carrots: *1 g protein, 2 g fiber, 35 calories*

Dinner
**Steak à la Chimichurri, Chimichurri, Chimichurri Churri!
(recipe, page 295)**
With Totally Nutty Sweet Potatoes (recipe, page 308)
42 g protein, 6 g fiber, 588 calories
Add 1 cup steamed broccoli: *5 g protein, 4 g fiber, 54 calories*

FRIDAY

Breakfast
Milky Oats with Strawberries, Hemp Seeds, and Peanut Butter
(recipe, page 241)
25 g protein, 7 g fiber, 520 calories

Snack
1 apple with 1 oz cheddar cheese
7 g protein, 4 g fiber, 209 calories

Lunch
1 slice whole grain toast topped with ½ avocado, mashed, and
¼ cup goat cheese
½ cup plain nonfat Greek yogurt topped with ½ cup
blackberries
27 g protein, 14 g fiber, 478 calories

Dinner
Let's treat ourselves to dinner at . . .
Olive Garden: Herb-Grilled Salmon served with broccoli
49 g protein, 9 g fiber, 495 calories

SATURDAY

Breakfast
Más Macho Nacho Supreme (recipe, page 258)
27 g protein, 10 g fiber, 485 calories

Snack
Bowl (1½ cups) of Oat O's cereal with ½ cup skim milk and
¼ cup blueberries
9 g protein, 5 g fiber, 225 calories

Lunch
Busy day! Let's hit the drive-thru at . . .
Wendy's: Large Chili + Caesar Side Salad
30 g protein, 13 g fiber, 580 calories

Dinner
Open Sesame Chicken and Veggies Stir-fry with Citrus Brown Rice (recipes, page 265 and 267)
34 g protein, 7 g fiber, 498 calories

Chapter 4

The Six Simple Secrets of Better Health

Here's What Your Body REALLY Needs Today

Once we come to see our midlife bodies for what they truly are—upgraded models that need better fuel to function optimally—then we can set about the process of tweaking our diets to get enough of the foods we need. Now that we know food impacts us differently as we get older, we can make better choices and ensure our bodies stay lean, fit, and in the best health possible for decades to come.

In this chapter, we'll take an in-depth look at the foods you need more of, a few you might want to eat less of, and why it's so important to pack your days with the fat-burning, muscle-protecting, life-giving nutrients you need.

The key word in the Whole Body Reset is consistency: How your body functions isn't dictated by what you eat on any given day, but what you eat consistently, day in and day out. In fact, rather than thinking of this as a "diet," think of it as a pattern of eating: Your simple goal is to select foods that deliver the nutrients your body needs.

Of course, as we learned in the previous chapter, our bodies don't necessarily absorb nutrients the way they once did. And yet, our bodies need those nutrients—the vitamins, minerals, and other plant nutrients—more than ever. That's why the information in this chapter is crucial. The more you can find your way to meeting these six secrets of health, the better you're going to feel over the long haul. And the long haul is what we're aiming for!

SIMPLE HEALTH SECRET #1
Eat 25–30 Grams of Quality Protein at Each Meal

"Most Americans eat enough protein." That's what the U.S. Department of Agriculture claims, and, technically, that's true. But imagine going through your entire day without drinking a drop of fluid, and then guzzling a gallon jug of water at dinnertime. You'd still be meeting the commonly recommended eight glasses a day, but you'd be going through most of your day feeling pretty fatigued and dehydrated. And you'd spend a lot of your night running to the bathroom.

Well, that's not unlike what happens to the average American when it comes to protein. The typical American diet looks like a tiny bit of protein at breakfast (milk in your cereal, maybe an egg or two); a bit more at lunch (a turkey sandwich perhaps); and then a huge infusion of protein (a steak or a couple of pork chops) at dinner. All told, we may consume an average of about 90 grams of protein a day, which is about what we need. But about two thirds of that typically comes at dinnertime.

And as we've shown, our bodies need 25 to 30 grams of protein—generally 25 grams for women, 30 for men—at each meal to keep the process of protein biosynthesis cranking along. Overeating protein at dinner doesn't help, because our bodies may only be able to use about 30 grams of protein at a time when at rest (although after exercise, our muscles are able to use more—up to 40 grams according to one study). So unless you just came back from the gym, a lot of that extra nighttime protein—while delicious and satisfying—won't be used to support your muscles. It'll be used to make more belly fat.

And speaking of calories—you'll notice we haven't made "cutting calories" a big part of this program. While the Whole Body Reset focuses more on increasing nutrition than on cutting calories, reducing junk calories is one area where a high-protein breakfast can help us. Several small studies[1] have found that increasing protein intake leads to an overall reduction in hunger, which means you won't be as tempted to grab something unhealthy. Protein also requires the body to expend more calories in digestion than carbs or fats do—a process known as "thermogenesis."[2] So why wouldn't you want this junk-food-suppressing power working its magic all day long?

You'll notice in Secret #1 a Q word—*quality*—snuck in before "protein." What's that about? Well, it's possible to eat lots of protein but still not get the essential muscle-building nutrients you need. What you're looking for are "complete" proteins.

A "complete" protein is one that delivers all nine "essential" amino acids—that is, those our bodies can't make. Amino acids are the building blocks of proteins, and research has indicated that, when it comes to building and maintaining muscle, leucine—one of the nine—may be the most important of these compounds.[3]

"It seems as though you need about three grams of leucine in a meal to really trigger the whole series of metabolic steps that turn on protein synthesis," says Doug Paddon-Jones, Sheridan Lorenz Distinguished Professor in Aging and Health at the Department of Nutrition and Metabolism, University of Texas Medical Branch. Paddon-Jones conducts studies on how different types and doses of protein affect muscle maintenance in people of different age groups. In one study, his team found that 4 ounces of lean beef, which contains approximately 30 grams of protein and 3 grams of leucine, boosted protein synthesis by 50 percent in both young and older adults.[4] Meanwhile, a separate review of studies found that leucine "significantly improves" sarcopenia in older adults.[5] And a short-term trial found that leucine, not total protein content, was the primary determinant of muscle protein anabolic response in healthy older women.[6]

That's important to note: While leucine does exist in plant foods, it's much more plentiful in animal products such as dairy, eggs, beef, and fish.[7] That's why these foods play a significant role in the Whole Body Reset—okay, that and the fact that most of us love to eat them. Animal proteins deliver all the essential amino acids. Plant-based sources also tend to be lower in lysine and methionine, two other essential amino acids.

But vegetarians and vegans have plenty of choices, too. Some plants—among them soy, buckwheat, quinoa, and hempseed—are complete proteins. Half a block of tofu yields about 2 grams of leucine, which will give you a solid start on your quest to reach at least 3 grams per meal. Otherwise, complete proteins can usually be formed by pairing grains, nuts, and seeds with a legume (peanuts, peas, dried beans, lentils). Many of our traditional vegetarian dishes happen to be exactly this combination: pita and hummus, corn and black bean salad, whole wheat toast with peanut butter. (You'll find a list of leucine-rich foods in the Muscle-Building Foods for Vegans table, on page 73.)

For vegans and vegetarians, eating plants in these combinations is critical. You may have read that the body can store proteins from different plant sources, so that as long as you eat an array of proteins throughout the day, you're fine.

"That's nonsense," says Paddon-Jones.

While our muscle-maintenance system is always humming along at some level, it can only kick in fully once it gets a jump start from the full complement of amino acids it needs. The idea that the body can store different types of amino acids and somehow put them together at the end of the day originated with a piece written in a medical journal in 1994.[8] In the report, researchers speculated that because a certain amino acid, lysine, is stored in muscle, perhaps the body could be capable of storing and combining amino acids during the course of the day. But much of that speculation was based partly on rat and pig studies, and no research on humans has actually shown this to be true, according to Paddon-Jones. In fact, his most recent studies have debunked this long-held myth—and helped lay out a blueprint for people who want to pursue a vegan diet.

"Rice and beans is a thing for a reason," he adds. "People worked this out a thousand years ago." Properly combined vegetable proteins are critical if you want to stimulate protein muscle synthesis and maintain muscle as you age. Think of the individual amino acids as essential bricks in a wall. "If you lack a complete set of bricks, you can't build that wall. The body can store as much fat and carbohydrate as you need, but it can't do that with protein. So the ability to use protein to build muscle depends on eating complementary proteins."

If you primarily eat a plant-based, vegetarian diet, it makes sense then to incorporate eggs and dairy into most meals to get all the complete protein you need. If you are vegan, you'll need to take extra care to get large amounts of plant protein throughout the day, especially from leucine-rich foods such as tofu and seitan.

Vegetarian, vegan, or not, you may also want to consider adding a plant-based protein mix—in powdered form added to a milk alternative or as a ready-to-drink beverage—to your diet. Look for mixes that are "complete" proteins—a mix of various plant sources such as pea, soy, and rice protein.

In fact, protein shakes and mixes are a great idea in general, says Paddon-Jones. Studies show that whey protein, derived from milk, may be the single best protein source for older people who want to retain muscle or rebuild muscle they've lost.

"A lot of people point to whey as one of the best options because it has a high amount of leucine," says Paddon-Jones. "Think of whey protein as a leucine-delivery system that comes in chocolate." You can easily find a variety of protein supplements that include powdered protein as well as liquid protein options that range from whey to plant-based, in either plain or flavored; they're typically found in the health food or health supplement section of your supermarket or drug store. The powdered or liquid proteins can be made into shakes or incorporated into foods such as oatmeal and baked goods. Or go the Italian route: Ricotta cheese is made primarily from whey protein and can turn your pizza or pasta into a protein-delivery system. Served chilled with berries, ricotta cheese also makes a pretty nice dessert.

Note: Whey protein powders come in two types: "concentrate" and "isolate." Whey concentrate is less expensive, but if you tend toward lactose sensitivity, choose whey isolate, which has had the lactose removed. Additionally, be sure to read the labels: Some protein supplements, especially protein bars and ready-to-drink mixes, are high in added sugars. (Use the Magic Supermarket Label Decoder formula in Chapter 8 to evaluate a quality product.) And, because protein powders are considered a supplement, they're not regulated by the FDA—meaning you don't always know what's in them. You can get an idea of how pure your product is by looking it up at cleanlabelproject.org.

TOP FOODS: Fish and shellfish; eggs (in moderation); poultry; nuts, seeds, and nut butters; lean meat; complete vegetable proteins, including soy, buckwheat, quinoa, and hempseed; combinations of grains and legumes that supply complete proteins; protein mixes and shakes (see Appendix 1, starting on page 341, for a more complete list of high-protein foods).

SIMPLE HEALTH SECRET #2
Enjoy Fortified Dairy Foods 2–3 Times a Day

Yes, you would like cheese on that. And whipped cream on top? Go for it.

As a source of complete protein, dairy is hard to beat. And as we get older, the benefits of milk, cheese, yogurt, and other forms of dairy only multiply.

That's due in part to dairy's protein punch—it's particularly high in leucine—but also to the many other nutrients it delivers, particularly calcium, magnesium, and vitamin D—all nutrients that our bodies have difficulty absorbing from food as we age,[9] and all of which help to keep us healthy and strong. In one study of older women, higher consumption of milk, yogurt, and cheese was associated with greater muscle mass and greater grip strength.[10]

Calcium

Chances are, you already understand the role that calcium plays in promoting strong bones: Studies suggest that approximately one in two women and as many as one in four men aged fifty and older will break a bone due to osteoporosis. In fact, 99 percent of the calcium in our bodies is found in our bones and teeth. And that helps to explain why it's so hard to get from food: Unless you're a giant living at the top of a beanstalk, you're probably not in the habit of grinding up bones to make your bread. Calcium comes from dairy, of course, plus nondairy sources such as leafy greens like broccoli and kale, soybeans, and the tiny bones we unknowingly ingest whenever we eat fish like sardines, canned salmon, or anchovies.

Calcium plays a key role in muscle maintenance, and it promotes heart health by helping to regulate blood pressure and blood clotting.[11]

But can't we just take a calcium supplement? Talk with your doctor about calcium supplements, but in general, studies on the effects of supplements have been inconclusive. Many doctors generally recommend we get our vitamins and minerals from foods rather than pills, if for no other reason than nutrition is an inexact science and whole foods provide a variety of nutrients that work synergistically to keep us healthy; it's not clear if a mineral like calcium works as effectively on its own as it does when ingested in combination with the other nutrients found in dairy and other foods.[12]

Magnesium

This often-overlooked mineral, found in dairy products, helps muscles and nerves function, assists in controlling blood sugar and blood pressure, and may play a role in preventing depression and Alzheimer's and preventing and managing diabetes. Yet magnesium doesn't get the marquee status of many other nutrients—in fact, most dairy products don't even mention this nutrient on their labels, even though they're all rich in it.

There are plenty of dietary sources of magnesium, yet most of us don't eat enough of them: nuts and seeds, beans, brown rice, and whole grain cereals among them. But if you're getting dairy several times a day, chances are you'll be meeting your daily allowance for this crucial nutrient—something nearly half of all Americans currently fail to do.

Vitamin D

Calcium and vitamin D go hand in hand, but—you may be surprised to learn—not naturally. Check out that milk carton in your refrigerator. On the ingredients label, you'll probably find "milk" and "vitamin D3." Maybe the label says "fortified." That's because by law, vitamin D must be added to milk. It's hard to get vitamin D from food sources other than those fortified with the vitamin, which is why the Whole Body Reset stresses "fortified" dairy. (Breakfast cereals are another food commonly fortified with vitamin D.)

Ideally, we'd each get at least 600 International Units (IUs) daily (and at least 800 after age seventy). Unfortunately, vitamin D is hard to find in adequate amounts in food; the average American diet yields about 274 IUs a day. The best sources, besides dairy and fortified foods, are fatty fish like salmon, mackerel, and sardines (vitamin D is stored in the fat) and Portobello mushrooms exposed to UV light. All healthy foods, but how many mackerel-and-mushroom-exposed-to-UV-light sandwiches have you eaten this week?

You've probably also heard that we can convert sunshine into vitamin D. That's true, to a certain point. But as we age, it gets harder for our bodies to manufacture vitamin D from the sun. That's partly because the skin's ability to synthesize vitamin D declines with age. We also tend to spend less time outdoors than we did when we were kids. Plus, D is fat-soluble, meaning it tends to be stored in belly fat. And when it's sequestered there, it's not available for use elsewhere in our bodies. A Korean study looked at the relationship between visceral fat and vitamin D and found that in women over the age of fifty, the more visceral fat they had, the lower their levels of vitamin D.

People of color are at special risk. In a 2006 report, 42 percent of Americans overall were D deficient, but the rate escalates to 63 percent for Hispanics and 82 percent for African Americans.

Because as we age we're manufacturing less vitamin D from the sun, we need more dietary vitamin D than our younger peers. One study showed that older adults with lower concentrations of vitamin D in their blood were twice as likely to suffer muscle loss over the ensuing three years; another study found that later in life, people with less vitamin D were at higher risk of having to enter a nursing home.[13] Other studies have shown that as vitamin D levels decline, risk of Parkinson's, Alzheimer's, and cognitive impairment rise. Vitamin D also serves as an air-traffic controller for calcium, essential for bone health: In one study of adults fifty and older, all of whom had recently fractured bones, 43 percent were deficient in both calcium and vitamin D. If you're low on vitamin D—and you probably are—ask your doctor about taking a daily supplement of 800 to 1000 IU.

Now, you might worry a bit about bloating from all this dairy, especially if you're lactose intolerant. But lactose—the natural sugar in dairy—is primarily found in milk, cottage cheese, and sugary milk products like ice cream. Hard cheese is very low in lactose: A cup of milk may have 12 to 13 grams of lactose, while cheddar and Swiss cheeses have less than one tenth of a gram. And yogurt and kefir are generally lower in lactose and well-tolerated by people with sensitivities. Because they are both fermented, they provide the added benefit of helping to support a healthy gut microbiome. (You'll read more about the importance of gut health on page 81.) So look for lactose-free milks, and in the meantime experiment with other dairy products to see which cause you issues and which you can enjoy at any time.

TOP FOODS: Milk, yogurt, and kefir fortified with vitamin D, cheese, cottage cheese, and whey-based protein smoothies (see page 127 for a list of dairy products).

SIMPLE HEALTH SECRET #3
Eat Colorful Fruits and Vegetables at Every Meal and Snack

Oh, you knew this part was coming, didn't you: The part where we tell you to eat more fruits and vegetables. Yes, and any diet plan that doesn't include heaping portions of produce should immediately be filed away as a snake-oil cure.

While all vegetables are good for you—assuming they're not coated with breading or deep-fried in oil—it helps to think of dark, leafy greens as the alpha veggies. Each day should include at least one helping—a small side salad or a ½ cup serving of cooked green vegetables—ensuring that you have a dietary source of the B vitamin folate. Folate also plays a crucial role in battling dementia, hearing loss, and depression in mature adults.[14] In a study of postmenopausal women, those who were overweight averaged 12 percent less folate in their blood than normal-weight women; those who were obese had 22 percent less.

Many leafy greens—broccoli, kale, brussels sprouts, arugula, cabbage, collards, and watercress—are also cruciferous vegetables (so named because the shape of their flowers, which have four petals, resembles a cross). Many root vegetables like turnips, radish, and rutabaga are also cruciferous. Studies show that these vegetables have a particularly powerful effect on our microbiome, helping to stabilize it and granting us improved immunity by lowering inflammation[15] levels.

Green is just one color. Variety is key: Scientists have identified more than 25,000 different phytonutrients ("phyto" = plant) in various plant foods, and these nutrients play a variety of different roles in reducing the incidence and progression of disease. The more plant foods we eat—colorful vegetables as well as fruits—the more we reap the benefits of these phytonutrients. Aim for 1½ to 2½ cups of vegetables a day.

In fact, while you should make a habit of reaching for a piece of fruit two to four times a day, try to make a particular effort to incorporate berries. Berries are among the fruits highest in fiber: One cup of raspberries gives you 8 grams of fiber, a cup of cantaloupe gives you just 1.4 grams. And berries may help keep both your body and your brain young and agile. One study found that those who

ingested the highest amounts of blueberries and strawberries reduced their cognitive age by up to two and a half years.

And we don't necessarily think of fruits and vegetables as muscle-
builders, but researchers are finding that more produce means more
muscle, especially as we age. For example, how would you like an
additional 3.6 pounds of lean, healthy muscle? That's how much
older people who ate lots of potassium-rich produce in one study
had, compared to their peers who ate only half as much potassium.
Another study showed that the more produce an older man consumes (fruits, vegetables, or a combination of the two), the lower his
risk of sarcopenia. The same study linked greater fruit consumption
among women to a lowered risk of muscle loss. These findings are
likely due to the fact that fruits and vegetables help to reduce inflammation,[16] and inflammation is muscle's enemy.[17] Researchers have
also discovered an association between higher levels of dietary vitamin C intake and greater muscle mass—more reasons to enjoy citrus fruits as well as berries, bell peppers, kiwi, cauliflower, tomatoes,
and the mighty broccoli. Keep it up and you'll see quick payoffs:
One small study of adults sixty-five and older found that those who
increased their fruit and vegetable intake from two to five portions
a day showed greater grip strength after sixteen weeks.[18]

TOP FOODS: All colorful vegetables and fruits, but especially dark,
leafy greens (lettuce, spinach, kale), cruciferous vegetables (broccoli,
cauliflower, brussels sprouts, arugula, cabbage, collards, watercress),
red and orange vegetables (carrots, squash, red peppers, tomatoes),
berries, tree fruits (apples, pears, cherries), and citrus (oranges,
grapefruit, lemons, limes) (see Appendix 1 for lists of colorful fruits
and veggies).

SIMPLE HEALTH SECRET #4
Aim for at Least 5 Grams of Fiber at Each Meal

Chances are, you don't eat enough fiber.

In fact, the average American eats about 15 grams of fiber a day—that's about the amount you'd find in a cup of black beans, or two cups of bran flakes, or three oat bran muffins, or five bananas, or ten carrots, or thirteen cups of popcorn.

That may seem like a lot of fiber, but it's not. In fact, it's about half of what experts believe we need to eat daily to ensure good health, and a leaner, fitter body. One study looked at the dietary habits of middle-aged women; when the researchers followed up twenty months later, they found that every additional gram of fiber the subjects ate correlated with a half a pound less in total weight, and a quarter percent less fat. The study[19] suggests that increasing fiber may have been the cause of that weight loss. If accurate, that means that if you went from eating 15 grams a day like the average American to eating 30 grams a day, you could drop 7.5 pounds, regardless of exercise levels or calorie reduction.

How can that be? Well, here's one explanation: Fiber can help block calorie absorption. A study found that people who ate the recommended daily allowance of fiber in the form of whole grains reduced their overall calorie balance by about 100 calories per day compared to people who ate refined grains, thanks to a combination of reduced calorie absorption and increased metabolism.

Pretty nifty trick, huh? Another long-term study followed African Americans and Hispanic Americans for five years and found that those who ate the most fiber had the lowest accumulation of belly fat.[20]

But how to get those extra grams? Fruits and vegetables are excellent sources of fiber, but chomping twenty carrots a day does not sound like a fun or sustainable eating plan. And a glass of a fiber supplement isn't going to cut it: Fiber supplements alone were ineffective at helping shed weight, according to one large study. The key is to pack our diet with fiber from a variety of grains, beans, and other plant foods.

And beans are efficient muscle-builders as well: When the Cleveland Clinic polled dietitians about their most-recommended sources of protein, Greek yogurt, eggs, and wild salmon were predictably in the top four. But their number one recommendation: beans, lentils, and split peas. Legumes provide protein and fiber; they even contain modest amounts of the crucial muscle-building amino acid leucine. And, like leafy greens, they're high in the B vitamin folate: In one study of older people with diabetes, the higher a person's folate levels, the greater their leg strength and grip strength.

To get the amount you need to keep your digestive system in top form, eat a whole grain and two servings of vegetables or fruit at each meal. Then top that off with high-fiber snacks: nuts, beans, fruits, and whole grain crackers throughout the day. See Chapter 14 for some yummy and easy ideas.

TOP FOODS: Whole wheat pasta, bread, tortillas, and crackers; oats; brown rice; quinoa; kasha; barley; beans; lentils; vegetables such as potatoes (with the skins on), brussels sprouts, peas, broccoli, and corn; and fruits, especially berries and tree fruits such as apples and pears (see tables in Appendix 1 for a list of high-fiber foods).

SIMPLE HEALTH SECRET #5
Enjoy More Healthy Fats

If you've been trying to lose weight by eating less fat, we have six key words of advice: *Stop trying to eat less fat.*

In fact, look at each meal as a chance to consume some healthy fats, between 15 and 30 grams per meal. That means some guacamole on your tacos, some olive oil on your salad, and—yes—some

2% or even whole milk with your cereal. In fact, there are three types of healthy fats you should be enjoying more of:

1. **Dairy fats.** Wow, really? Yep, it's true. While you've been told to avoid saturated fats from whole-fat dairy, the real deal is more complicated: Fat from dairy may offer protection from cardio-vascular disease, according to a recent study. Plus—and you may want to sit down with your curds and whey for this one—it turns out that full-fat dairy has been linked to a *reduced* risk of obesity. That's partly because of all the nice, healthy protein, vitamins, and minerals that dairy comes with, but it may also be because the creamy fats are satisfying and reduce the desire to snack later on. (But that's full-fat milk, cheeses, and unsweetened yogurts; it doesn't mean you can max out on frozen yogurt or ice cream every evening. Sugar changes everything.)

2. **Omega-3 fatty acids.** These healthy fats have been shown to play a role in reducing belly fat and in promoting muscle preservation in older adults.[21] You'll find them primarily in fatty fish such as salmon, mackerel, sardines, and tuna—and eating fish even twice a week affords these benefits. But again, it's from food. Before you spend your hard-earned money on supplements, stop and consider the science: While studies link foods rich in this fat to a lower risk of cardiovascular disease, results of studies assessing omega-3 pills have been mixed.[22] It's possible that, to be effective, omega-3 needs to be taken in combination with some of the other nutrients found in the omega-3-rich fish, soybeans, walnuts, flax seeds, or chia seeds.

3. **Fruit and nut oils.** Olive oil is the go-to here (yep, olives are a fruit, as are avocados), because so much research has been conducted on it. Indeed, recent animal studies have shown that extra-virgin olive oil may reduce the risk of dementia by flushing out the pro-

teins that gum up the communications channels between brain cells. The secret is in the olive's special nutrient, a polyphenol called oleocanthal. You know that bite you get at the back of your throat when you taste a really good olive oil? The oleocanthal causes it—it's a sign that your brain is getting a boost! (You'll read more about this secret nutrient on page 109.) To get an olive oil that's rich in this nutrient, always select "extra-virgin," and look for a brand that comes in a dark green bottle or tin; these packages help protect the oil from sun damage.

The type of fat in your diet impacts the type of fat in your muscles; opting for monounsaturated fats is like hitting the Tin Man with a healthy oil can, leading to healthier, better-functioning muscles. Nuts, seeds, avocado, and olives are also excellent sources of vitamin E which, like other antioxidants, help to protect the health of bodily tissues. Another crucial nutrient healthy fats deliver: magnesium, which is found in high levels in pumpkin seeds, almonds, cashews, and peanuts. One study found higher blood levels of magnesium were associated with stronger grip strength and leg-muscle power in older adults.

TOP FOODS: Seafood, oils (olive, safflower, peanut, sesame), nuts, seeds, avocado, and olives

SIMPLE HEALTH SECRET #6
Don't Drink Your Calories (or Chemicals)

Ever hear that term "recharge your batteries"? It's not a metaphor: Your body really does have batteries—untold trillions of them, actually. Those batteries are known as mitochondria, and they're found in cells throughout the body. Fully functioning mitochondria may help prevent the onset of Alzheimer's, heart disease, Parkinson's, and diabetes, among other common ills.[23] And in addition to eating good food and getting enough sleep, there's a third way to recharge them: Drinking enough water.

In fact, studies suggest that as our cells expand with proper fluid intake, the mitochondria may become more active, possibly increasing the rate of fat-burning[24] and helping to lead to weight loss.

But when it comes to fluids, extra calories can be trouble. A significant source of empty calories in the American diet is beverages. Soda, iced teas, specialty coffee drinks, "sports" drinks, oversized smoothies and shakes, even fruit juices—they are, for the most part, loaded with sugar. And this idea ought to make you rethink your next café mocha: Liquid sugars move through the digestive tract more quickly than solids, allowing more of them to enter the colon, where they literally can feed precancerous growths called polyps.[25]

The Whole Body Reset avoids calorie-laced drinks as well as diet sodas, which have been shown to increase appetite and, in some studies, have been linked to an increase in the risk of heart disease, dementia, and stroke. They may also hurt our microbiome,[26] which is really, other than skin, our first-line defense against infection and oh-so-important for continuing to absorb nutrients from the food we eat. Instead, the Whole Body Reset promotes increased consumption of water, unsweetened tea and coffee, and dairy. That's because drinking more fluids will lead to better overall health, and even weight loss. In one study of adults aged fifty-five to seventy-five who were on calorie-controlled diets, those who drank 17 ounces of water thirty minutes before each daily meal lost on average about 4.5 pounds more than those who didn't drink water beforehand.[27]

But as we've already stated, drinking substantial amounts of water and other calorie-free drinks reduces your risk of obesity.

About Your Drinking Habit . . .

Actually, it could be your lack of a drinking habit that's the problem. One study found that more than half of adults in the United States don't drink enough water. And by the time we reach sixty, we tend to drink less—about two fewer cups of liquid every day than younger people do.

Plus, being properly hydrated helps to aid in the absorption of nutrients—another concern as we get older.

We have all sorts of excuses not to drink water. We're too busy; we forget; we prefer the taste of sweet drinks; we're not so thirsty (which may be true—our thirst sensation tends to diminish with age). Which brings us back to your drinking habit: Start now by accompanying every meal with a big glass of water, sparkling water, or unsweetened coffee or tea. You'll start another healthy habit for life.

TOP CALORIE-FREE DRINKS: Water (still or sparkling, plain or flavored with fruit slices), unsweetened tea and coffee

Muscle-Building Foods for Vegans

Leucine is plentiful in animal products, but when eating a plants-only diet, it's harder to get the 3 grams of leucine per meal we need to build and maintain muscle. Here are the best vegan sources (in order of leucine content):

FOOD	SERVING	LEUCINE (IN GRAMS)
Seitan	3½ oz	5.9
Tempeh	1 cup	2.4
Soy protein powder	1 scoop	2
Tofu	1 cup	1.8
Sunflower seeds	1 tbsp	1.7
Sesame seeds	¼ cup	1
Edamame (frozen)	1 cup	0.8
Pumpkin seeds	¼ cup	0.7
Hemp seeds	3 tbsp	0.7
Navy beans	½ cup	0.6
Kidney beans	½ cup	0.6
Chickpeas	½ cup	0.5
Almonds	¼ cup	0.5
Peanuts	¼ cup	0.5
Pasta, dry	½ cup	0.4

Sources: U.S. Department of Agriculture National Agricultural Library (www.nal.usda. gov/sites/www.nal.usda.gov/files/leucine.pdf); veganhealth.org

— ACTION STEP #4 —

While protein is essential, one particular source of protein—dairy foods—provides a nutritional one-two punch. When we eat dairy, we're also getting a number of crucial vitamins and minerals that are hard to find in other foods. Name four dairy foods you can add this week to increase your overall intake, and where they might fit into your diet (for example, cheese—on my pasta). For a cheat sheet, see the Complete Whole Body Reset Mix 'N' Match Meal Maker in Appendix 1.

1. _____

2. _____

3. _____

4. _____

Chapter 5

The Inside Story of Your Gut

What Exactly IS Belly Fat, and Where Does It Come From?

At the beginning of Chapter 1, I asked you to look down at your belly.

You probably think you know that belly pretty good—its rolls, its creases, whether you're sporting an innie or an outie. But most of us actually know very little about our belly fat.

For example, did you know that it used to be somewhere else?

Think of yourself back when you were a baby. You've seen the pictures, how you used to have fat all over the place—chubby cheeks, chubby thighs, even chubby wrists. As we grow into our teens and twenties and thirties, that fat spreads throughout our bodies, often gathering in pleasing ways, right where we want it to be. But as we get older, the fat begins to shift again, consolidating itself around our midsections. So that expanding waistline isn't a mark of sloth, gluttony, or any of the other deadly sins. It's just some old friends who have moved into a different neighborhood.

Weird, right?

But that's not the only strange fact about your belly. You see, belly fat isn't just sitting there, mocking you as you try to button your jeans. While it may seem stubborn and unmoving, belly fat is, in fact, tremendously active.

It is very, very busy trying to ruin your health.

Why Belly Fat Makes Your Whole Body Angry

There's a sort of triad of unhealthy aging—an "Axis of Evil," as George W. Bush might put it. It's the combination of diminished muscle quality, increased inflammation, and expanding belly fat. They're the Three Stooges of illness, each of them egging the other two on to greater and greater mischief. But in this confederacy of dunces, belly fat is the ringleader.

Belly fat cells are, in essence, miniature endocrine organs releasing hormones and other pesky chemicals into your body. Among them are inflammatory proteins called cytokines, which contribute to a number of inflammation-related problems. Harvard researchers have also found that visceral fat cells secrete higher levels of a molecule called RBP4, which increases insulin resistance, putting us at greater risk of diabetes and weight gain. Yes, belly fat causes you to gain belly fat.

The COVID-19 crisis laid this out for us clearly: In a study of how the stay-at-home orders impacted people, researchers in the journal *Obesity* found that 27.5 percent of the 7,753 people surveyed said they gained weight during the lockdown. But among people who were already obese, that number jumped to 33.4 percent. The more visceral fat you have, the harder it is to prevent future weight gain. Unless you make a change.

And we've already established that inflammation plays a role in reducing muscle volume.[1] Muscle happens to be very good at storing excess calories, so when we have less muscle, we have more free calories that can be turned into . . . wait for it . . . belly fat. So, more belly

Did You Say That My Belly Fat Is Making Me Fat?

Yes, we did. "Fat, especially belly fat, is a highly inflammatory tissue," says Dana DiRenzo, a rheumatologist and instructor of medicine at Penn Medicine in Philadelphia. Every day, your belly fat is creating and releasing inflammatory compounds with Bond-villain names such as interleukin 6 and tumor necrosis factor-alpha, DiRenzo explains. It's why lifestyle factors such as not sleeping well can cause weight gain; it's not just about calories, but about inflammation as well.

Remember, inflammation is a response to cell damage—and fat cells are the body's damsels in distress. They're bloated with triglycerides (a substance similar to diesel fuel) and as a result, they are very fragile and can easily burst and die. When they do, they trigger an inflammatory response as the immune system sends white blood cells to clean up the spilled fuel.

fat = more inflammation = less muscle = more belly fat. As belly-fat-inspired inflammation rises, our risk of just about everything increases:[2] Researchers at Kaiser Permanente found that those with the greatest levels of abdominal fat in their forties were nearly three times more likely to develop dementia in their seventies or eighties than those who had the least belly fat.[3]

Your Belly Is Changing on the Inside, Too

You can think of an expanding waistline as both the cause and the symptom of poor health. But there's even more mischief happening deep inside your gut.

As we age, the way our digestive system absorbs nutrients changes. It becomes harder and harder for us to get the vital nutrients we need from food, partly due to increased inflammation. And that creates a feedback loop—the bigger your belly, the more your digestive system struggles, Katherine Tucker, director of the Center for Population Health at the University of Massachusetts in Lowell, told me. Indeed, it helps to think of belly fat as one giant inflammation marker—the lower your inflammation, the smaller your belly, and vice versa. That's why belly fat is linked so directly to so many illnesses.

"Depending on your health, malabsorption issues can arise at different ages, but generally people should start being concerned about it after age fifty," says Tucker. The term "malabsorption" refers to the body's inability to turn all the good stuff in food into fuel the body can use.

Malabsorption happens partly because the contents of our stomachs change, as we begin to produce less stomach acid. But stomach acid is critical for digestion, particularly when it comes to extracting certain nutrients from food. Take vitamin B12. Found exclusively in animal foods, B12 is essential for producing healthy red blood cells and preserving nerve function. It also seems to play a role in preventing depression in older adults.[4] Research shows that while the vast

---

30

The number of different plants you should include in your diet every week, according to a multinational study of more than ten thousand people. Compared to people who ate fewer than ten different plants per week, those eating more than thirty performed significantly better in a battery of gut tests—the most notable being microbiome diversity.

majority of us eat enough B12-rich foods to meet our recommended daily allowance, as many as one in five older adults have gastric issues that may interfere with their ability to absorb B12.

Think back to that breakfast you and your child shared in Chapter 2. While you may have consumed the same amount of B12-rich egg protein, you may well have netted out at very different doses of this vitamin. Vitamins B6 and B2—both crucial to helping the body process protein and manage inflammation—are two other nutrients the older body may have difficulty absorbing, says Tucker.

But it's not just stomach acid levels that differentiate your gut from that of your child. With age, the very biology of our bellies changes.[5]

As infants, we inherit a diverse array of trillions of bacteria, located primarily in the digestive tract. These bacteria, known as the microbiome, are our best friends for life: They help digest food, manage inflammation, protect against disease, and perform dozens of other useful tasks. They are the ultimate live-in help.

But over the course of our lives, we don't necessarily treat our BFFs as well as we should. Stress,[6] poor diet (especially a lack of fiber), and the use of antibiotics and other medications damage the diverse ecosystem within our guts. Meanwhile, too much sugar and too many artificial chemicals (including artificial sweeteners) disrupt the balance of bacteria in our guts.[7] The bacteria that thrive in this disrupted environment play a role in increasing inflammation throughout our bodies, and the more unhealthy bacteria there are, the more they overwhelm the helpful bacteria that keep inflammation in check. Over time this disruption damages our gut, which may make it even more difficult for our bodies to absorb the vitamins and minerals we need from our otherwise nutritious and delicious eggs-and-toast breakfast. And an altered microbiome also seems to lead to excess calorie absorption—meaning you absorb more calories from food than a person with a healthier gut.[8]

Our gut microbiome plays a role in countless physiologic pro-

GUTSY DECISIONS
Foods that Spark—and Soothe—Inflammation

SPARK	SOOTHE
White bread: A diet low in fiber can allow unhealthy bacteria to gain the upper hand in your digestive system, contributing to a leaky gut, in which toxins are allowed to pass through into your body rather than being swept away by the digestive system.	**Whole grain bread:** As the body digests fiber, like that found in whole grains, it creates butyrate, a beneficial fatty acid with anti-inflammatory powers. Butyrate may help prevent neurological decline.
Deep fryers: Inflammation-causing compounds called advanced glycation end products (AGEs) are produced when meats and grains are cooked at high heat—think doughnuts, French fries, and fried chicken.	**Fruit bowls:** Dark-colored fruits as well as vegetables and beans contain polyphenols, plant compounds with antioxidant and anti-inflammatory properties.
Pudding: Most processed foods, especially desserts, are low in fiber, high in sugar, and packed with chemicals, all of which are bad for the gut. The more you cook at home with unprocessed food, the better.	**Yogurt:** Live-culture yogurts contain healthy bacteria called probiotics, which help keep the bad gut bacteria in check.
Bottled salad dressings: Look at the label of your favorite dressing. The first three ingredients are probably water, sugar, and soybean oil. Soybean and vegetable oils are high in omega-6 fatty acids—which we tend to eat a lot of. Make your own salad dressings with olive oil, lemon or vinegar, and spices.	**Big, colorful salads:** The vitamins, minerals, and phytonutrients found in fruits and vegetables help prevent cell damage via oxidative stress—in other words, they fight inflammation. There are hundreds of antioxidants, such as vitamins A, C, and E, as well as lycopene and selenium.

cesses throughout the body. A healthy gut is one that maintains a balance between good and bad bacteria. Imbalance might lead to trouble, as an "imbalanced" gut has been associated with metabolic diseases, pulmonary diseases, nervous system conditions, and Alzheimer's, among other disorders.

As changes in our digestive system and our microbiome make it harder for us to absorb and use the nutrients in our food, we've got to give our bodies the opportunity to pack in more and more nutrition with our meals, particularly the vitamins and minerals we're becoming resistant to. The Whole Body Reset is built around these crucial, life-giving nutrients.

The Care and Feeding of Your Belly

What your dysregulated little belly buggers crave is more fiber.

Fiber is the edible, but undigestible, parts of plants. Our early ancestors ate about 100 grams of fiber per day,[9] one researcher has estimated; the average American eats about 16.

That's a big drop-off, and it hasn't been kind to us. The more fiber you eat, the lower your risk of the six most deadly diseases known to humans: heart disease, cancer, chronic respiratory disease, stroke, Alzheimer's, and diabetes. Which makes you think: If it's indigestible, how can it make a difference to my health?

In part, it's because what's indigestible to you isn't necessarily indigestible to your little friends, the microbiome. The billions of bacteria in your gut feast on these morsels, breaking them down into what are called short-chain fatty acids, compounds that disperse into the blood stream and help to quell chronic inflammation. The Mayo Clinic recommends at least 3 grams of fiber at breakfast but says 5 grams or more is even better. The piece of whole grain toast you ate provided you with less than half of that.

So while protein is job one in the Whole Body Reset, fiber plays a crucial role as well. In the coming pages, you'll discover not just how this program can help you drop pounds, but how the Whole Body Reset can help turn around the direction of your health, and your life.

— ACTION STEP #5 —

Fiber helps maintain gut health and, in doing so, lowers our risk of disease, helps our bodies maintain muscle, and even encourages weight loss. But the average American gets only about half the fiber needed each day.

Let's tackle that problem right now. Name three fiber-rich foods you've eaten in the past week and three you can add this week to increase your overall intake. (For a cheat sheet, see the Complete Whole Body Reset Mix 'N' Match Meal Maker in Appendix 1.)

Last Week	**Next Week**
1. _____	_____
2. _____	_____
3. _____	_____

Chapter 6

How the Whole Body Reset Can Help Fight Disease and Save Your Life

(Over and Over Again)

You'll Not Only Look Better, You'll Live Better, Too!

If the Whole Body Reset seems to appeal to our vanity, that's okay. There's nothing wrong with wanting to look our best. But a sleeker body is just the cherry on top of this program, because it's likely that your greatest and most lasting impact will be on your health, your longevity, and your overall quality of life.

That's partly because simply by seizing control of your food and your weight, you automatically seize more control over your health as well. You've been told this a bazillion times, but it bears repeating, this time with a series of definitive reports to prove it: One looked at 189 studies conducted with 4 million people on four continents and found that being overweight or obese increased your risk of death[1] from all causes combined. In another study, researchers followed older people (average age: sixty-three) for twenty-four years and found that even accounting for preexisting health conditions and lifestyle choices like smoking, being obese was independently responsible for a significantly higher death rate.[2]

Stop age-related weight gain and muscle loss, and you're taking a huge step toward saving your own life. But you already knew that, didn't you?

Well, you might not know that eating more protein—specifically, more plant protein—was linked to lower risk of death from any cause, including cancer and heart disease,[3] according to a review of thirty-two separate studies.

Okay, so this program can help you live longer, and it can help you live leaner. But those are just two legs of the overall health stool. The third leg is to live healthier—to have an active, enjoyable life brimming with rewarding adventures and fulfilling relationships. In this chapter, we'll explain how the food and fitness components of this plan have been shown to reduce our risk of a remarkable number of health conditions and concerns, and can reduce our risk of pain, disability, and disease. Think inflammation, colds, flu, even the coronavirus. Think diabetes, heart disease, and dementia (which is covered in the next chapter). And more. Just look at all the Whole Body Reset can do for you.

You'll Slow "Inflammaging"

As grown-ups, the changes in our gut microbiome, the reduced levels of muscle, and the inability of our bodies to fully absorb nutrients are all related to one massive bodily insult: chronic inflammation. We've mentioned its role in weight gain in earlier chapters, but more and more experts are looking at inflammation as the master manipulator of age-related health woes. In fact, there's even a relatively new term for the increase in inflammation as we get older: inflammaging.[4]

Think about when you catch the flu and your body temperature rises to fight the virus. That's the result of inflammation. So is the redness and warmth that occur when an injury is healing; it's the process your body uses to provide the restorative chemicals and nutrients needed to help repair the damage. These are examples of "acute" inflammation: a temporary, helpful response to an injury or illness. Once the danger goes away, so does the inflammation.

"Chronic" inflammation, on the other hand, is a slow, creeping condition caused by a misfiring of the immune system that keeps your body in a constant, long-term state of high alert. Low-grade inflammation is linked to a multitude of diseases, from diabetes to cancer, but its effect on the immune system can be like a prank-ster who's constantly pulling the fire alarm. Your immune system responds, often inappropriately, attacking harmless invaders (think of how some people get allergic reactions to harmless substances, from pollen to peanuts) and even healthy body tissue. After years of chasing after all these false calls, the immune system gets exhausted and distracted, and hence less capable of responding properly when a real fire is unleashed.

"Over time, inflammation damages healthy cells," Roma Pahwa, a researcher for the National Institutes of Health who specializes in the inflammatory response, told AARP. Here's why: When cells are in distress, they release chemicals that alert the immune system. White blood cells then flood the scene, where they work to eat up bacteria, viruses, damaged cells, and debris from an infection or injury.

If the damage is too great, they call in a backup type of white blood cells known as neutrophils, which are the hand grenades of the immune system—they blow up everything in sight, healthy or not. Neutrophils have a short life span, but in chronic inflammation, they continue to be sent in long after the real threat is gone, causing damage to the healthy tissue that remains. The inflammation can start attacking the linings of your arteries or intestines, the cells in your liver and brain, or the tissues of your muscles and joints. This inflammation-caused cellular damage can trigger diseases like diabetes, cancer, dementia, heart disease, arthritis, and depression.

And because the inflammation is low grade, "its slow and secret nature makes it hard to diagnose in day-to-day life," Pahwa says. "You have no idea it's even happening until those conditions show symptoms."

By lowering chronic inflammation, you help to reduce the risk and impact of infectious diseases like COVID-19 as well as heart disease, diabetes, dementia, and more than one hundred other serious conditions.

A variety of things can trigger that low-grade inflammation, including genetics, diseases, and pollution. But age is the biggest contributor of all. It's not just the natural changes in our bodies, but the accumulation of challenges we've put ourselves through: years of stress, lack of exercise, poor sleep, late nights in smoky bars—the bad-for-you stuff adds up over the decades.

Some foods also play a role in increasing inflammation, and you can probably guess what they are. They're the same foods that everyone from your dentist to your cardiologist has warned you about. And that's no surprise, because gingivitis and sclerotic arteries are both inflammatory conditions. Foods high in sugar (yummy cakes and cookies and candy) or high in unhealthy fats (fried anything) top the list, as well as deli meats and processed foods that have been stripped of their natural fiber (white rice, potato chips, refined flour products such as white bread, pretzels, and pancakes). In a study following 2,735 people starting at age forty-nine for thirteen years, women who ate the most sugary foods and the least amount of fiber were 2.9 times as likely to die from inflammation-based diseases such as heart disease.[5]

Real food—food in its natural, unprocessed form—actually helps to fight inflammation, thanks to its vitamins, minerals, proteins, fiber, healthy fats, and phytochemicals. Phytochemicals, by the way, are the nutrients that give plants their bright colors—making blackberries black, blueberries blue, oranges orange, and red onions, um, purple. But as our bodies age, and we have difficulty processing many of these nutrients—specifically vitamins, minerals, protein, and phytochemicals—those foods become less effective in helping us battle inflammation. We may be fighting disease with the same lightsaber, but the batteries aren't fully charged.

So, inflammation makes it harder for the body to extract nutrients. A lack of nutrients causes an increase in inflammation. It's a punishing cycle, and it requires us to take greater care to ensure we're getting the nutrients we need to keep inflammation under control.

That's why the Whole Body Reset is packed with anti-inflammatory foods. A diet rich in polyphenols reduced inflammation and improved overall gut health in one small study of people sixty and older. Researchers have also recently discovered that the more fruits and vegetables older adults eat, the lower their degree of sarcopenia as they age. Polyphenols discourage inflammation. And inflammation is toxic to muscle. One study of obese older adults found a significant link between reduced lean muscle tissue and three markers of chronic inflammation.[6] And that, in turn, leads to more levels of fat (especially belly fat).

But when you build muscle, you lower inflammation. Imagine belly fat and skeletal muscle in an all-out tug-of-war: The more you have of one, the less you are likely to have of the other. In fact, muscle is a "major immune regulatory organ," according to a 2019 study.[7] And it does its best firefighting when we exercise, especially when we exercise the large muscles of the body, like the thighs and butt. (Think squats and stair climbing.) With lower inflammation, you lower the risk of chronic inflammatory diseases such as atherosclerosis, diabetes mellitus,[8] and insulin resistance. Exercise may even boost the immune system by improving gut health.

You're going to read about the "I" word—inflammation—throughout this chapter, and throughout this book. It really is, in many ways, the king of all our physical woes: the crown prince of cardiovascular disease, the duke of diabetes, the kaiser of cancer, and the emperor of Alzheimer's (which you'll read more about in the next chapter). By lowering chronic inflammation, you help to reduce the risk and impact of infectious diseases like COVID-19 as well as heart disease, diabetes, dementia, and more than a hundred other serious conditions, among them rheumatoid arthritis, celiac disease, psoriasis, Crohn's disease, Raynaud's disease, restless leg syndrome, ulcerative colitis, and endometriosis.

You'll Help Protect Yourself from Colds, Flu, and Coronaviruses

When we think of the immune system, we often think in terms of antibodies and white blood cells, stuff we learned about in junior high—and then read even more about during the COVID-19 crisis. And yes, one aspect of our immune system encompasses these little armies of intrepid defenders, traveling about our blood vessels, looking for some troublemaking virus or bacteria to tussle with. We don't necessarily associate the immune system with inflammation, but we should. Because while chronic inflammation can mess up a lot of things for us as we age, it also has the secondary effect of distracting and confusing the immune system, thereby hampering our ability to fight off disease. Consider this: Among 5,700 patients who were hospitalized for the coronavirus in the spring of 2020 in the New York City area, 34 percent had diabetes, 42 percent were obese, and 57 percent had high blood pressure, according to a study published in *the Journal of the American Medical Association (JAMA)*. A common factor for all three conditions is chronic inflammation, which causes your immune system to pump out white blood cells and chemical messengers, keeping your defenses actively engaged 24/7. As a result, when a viral infection, cold, or flu sets in, your immune system is already otherwise engaged. It may not be able to muster an appropriate response.

In addition to throwing a wet blanket on chronic inflammation, the Whole Body Reset can help you to keep your immune system healthy in several other ways:

❑ **By boosting fiber intake.** Fiber feeds the good bacteria in your gut. When you help keep the little buggers happy, they help keep your immune system functioning at its peak.[9]

❑ **By upping your beta-carotene.** Beta-carotene is what your body uses to create vitamin A, a crucial vitamin in the creation of several different immune cells. Orange foods (like carrots, cantaloupe, and sweet potatoes) and leafy greens (like spinach, romaine lettuce, and kale) are among the best sources.

❑ **By enjoying more cruciferous vegetables.** We've talked about these in earlier chapters, but they're a crucial part of any diet. Broccoli, cauliflower, and cabbage, among others, contain an amino acid called cysteine, which helps your body produce an antioxidant called glutathione, a powerful immune system regulator. In fact, why don't you just order the coleslaw and get all three of the above bullets taken care of in one meal?

❑ **By eating more fish.** Omega-3 fatty acids from oily fish such as sardines and salmon can cut inflammation in older adults, which means a healthier immune system.[10]

❑ **By increasing your vitamin C intake the right way.** Okay, you know that vitamin C is linked to immunity; you've seen those megadose vitamin C tablets in your local pharmacy, or perhaps come across those dissolvable packets you're supposed to drink down when you feel a slight cold coming on. But here's the thing: Some vitamins, like vitamin A, D, E, and K, are fat-soluble. That means you store them in your body. Others, like B vitamins and vitamin C, are not. Whatever your body can't use in the moment just flushes through your system and follows Nemo down the drain. That's why vitamin C throughout the day, consumed from natural sources like fruits and vegetables with each meal, is a far better choice than simply popping a supplement—or downing a big, calorie-laden glass of orange juice with breakfast—and thinking you've got it covered. (If you're an OJ fan, trade in the big morning glass for several small servings throughout the day to keep yourself covered and reduce that big sugar load.)

❑ **By providing you with more foods rich in zinc.** The protein that powers the Whole Body Reset also ensures that you'll be topped off in this important immunity nutrient. Beef, shellfish, pork, beans, and tofu are all rich in zinc.

❑ **By helping you build and maintain muscle.** When you improve immune system function and reduce inflammation, you don't just protect against viruses. You also give your body the ability to fend off other serious health threats—specifically cancer. Breast cancer patients who have high muscle mass have a greater chance of surviving the disease than those who have lower muscle mass, according to a study of 3,241 women (median age: fifty-four) with stage 2 or 3 breast cancer. And, in a study of men who had undergone a radical prostatectomy to treat prostate cancer, researchers found that those with the lowest levels of muscle were more likely to see a recurrence of the cancer and more likely to eventually die of the disease.

You'll Protect Yourself from Heart Disease

Cardiovascular health isn't a singular issue. It's a complex interchange of several factors: controlled blood pressure, a well-balanced cholesterol profile, and healthy blood vessels free of plaque buildup. Each of these pillars is essential to keeping your cardiovascular system in fine working order. (As is a strong heart muscle, which you can help to build with the exercise program in Chapter 12, Your Whole Body Fitness Plan.)

But as we've already pointed out, high blood pressure, high cholesterol, and plaque buildup in the arteries are all symptoms of the larger, underlying issue of inflammation. Indeed, a study showed that in people who had suffered a previous heart attack, reducing inflammation cut their risk of subsequent heart attack or stroke by 15 percent, even if their cholesterol levels stayed the same.

By following the nutritional recommendations in this book, you'll reduce inflammation and hence reduce your risk of heart disease. But you'll also . . .

❏ **Help to reduce your blood pressure.** One major contributor to our epidemic of high blood pressure is that so much of our food—particularly the prepackaged, processed stuff like sandwich meats and snacks—is too high in sodium (the mineral that boosts blood pressure) and too low in potassium (the mineral that helps lower it). In fact, if you think your blood pressure as a seesaw, sodium would sit on one end, looking to send it spiking into the sky. Potassium sits at the other end, trying to even it out. By reducing the junk food and eating whole, natural plants and proteins, you'll dramatically reduce sodium while boosting potassium and calcium. Calcium and potassium come readily in the form of dairy, and you'll also find potassium in fruits and vegetables, particularly bananas, grapefruit, oranges, avocados, zucchini, beans, and potatoes. And other foods you'll be enjoying on the Whole Body Reset—from probiotic-rich yogurt to fiber-filled almonds to nutrient-dense dark chocolate[11]—can play a role in keeping blood pressure in check.

❏ **Improve your cholesterol numbers and the health of your arteries.** Inflammation plays an enormous role in the health of your arteries, which is just one reason why loading your plate with a wide variety of colorful fruits and vegetables can make a big impact on whether or not your cardiologist gives you a passing grade. In a study involving 115 older adults (average age: sixty-three) who had metabolic conditions, those who ate 1 cup of blueberries each day for six months showed improved vascular function and higher levels of heart-healthy HDL cholesterol. The study's authors credited an antioxidant called anthocyanin, which is also found in cherries, blackberries and other red, purple, and blue foods. Betalain is another powerful plant pigment. It makes beets red, and in one study, supplementing with the compound resulted in lower levels of homocysteine—an amino acid that can damage the lining of the arteries—as well as improved levels of blood glucose and unhealthy LDL cholesterol. (It lowered blood pressure as well.)

❏ **Reduce your risk of stroke.** The same factors that endanger our hearts—unhealthy cholesterol, high blood pressure, stiffened arteries—put us at risk of stroke as well. And the same remedies that protect our hearts protect us from these terrifying brain attacks. For example, we know that fiber is good for our hearts—and food marketers know that you know, which is why they love, love, love putting those little red hearts on the packaging of their high-fiber breakfast cereals. But lift your fiber intake, and you also dramatically slash your risk of stroke, according to a review of studies from around the world. Another analysis of studies got even more specific: For every additional 10 grams of fiber you eat per day, you reduce your risk of stroke by 12 percent.[12]

But perhaps the most surprising way the Whole Body Reset protects your heart is by helping you grow and maintain muscle mass. In one study, high levels of muscular strength appear to protect men with high blood pressure from premature death.[13] And in another study of men (average age: forty-three), researchers found that among those with prehypertension, higher levels of muscular strength were associated with a reduced risk of developing full-blown hypertension in the ensuing years.[14] Muscle lowers your risks from metabolic syndrome, obesity, and inflammation as well.

You'll Bar the Door Against Diabetes

If type 2 diabetes (that is, dangerously high blood sugar) is a concern for you—and it should be, since one in six Americans ages forty-five to sixty-four and one in four over age sixty-five has the disease, and more than one in three American adults is prediabetic—then you should probably be thinking, "What's the single best nutritional step I can take to lower my risk?" The answer may be incredibly simple: Eat a protein-rich breakfast every day.

Let me repeat those final two words: Every day. Whether you're diabetic, prediabetic, or just never want to have the disease.

Researchers conducted a meta-analysis of studies encompassing more than 96,000 participants and discovered that for every day of the week you skip breakfast, your risk of diabetes grows bigger. Those who skipped one day a week had a greater risk than those who ate breakfast every day, those who skipped two days had a greater risk than those who skipped just one, and up the risk went to five days.[15] Each day that you wake up and decide something more important than breakfast is happening, your diabetes risk grows.

And a protein-rich breakfast has been shown to help control blood sugar levels in people with type 2 diabetes not just in the morning but during subsequent meals later in the day.[16]

Each day when you wake up, you make the choice. A protein-rich breakfast—the foundation of the Whole Body Reset—sets you on a path to retaining and building muscle, and muscle—by providing a storage space for blood sugar—plays an enormous role in helping to control diabetes. One study of 13,644 subjects found that those with the lowest percentage of muscle were 63 percent more likely to have diabetes than those with the highest percentage.[17]

But as we age, and begin to lose muscle, we have less storage space. Blood sugar builds up. And the body, frantic to manage this buildup of blood sugar, makes the second-best choice: It turns that excess blood sugar into belly fat.

Belly fat, as you know, increases inflammation. And diabetes is an inflammatory disease. So begins the vicious cycle in which our risks from diabetes—from blindness to organ failure to heart disease—just grow and grow.[18]

You'll Maintain Mobility and Reduce Your Risk of Falls and Broken Bones

When AARP surveyed adults fifty and older about their top health concerns, we got many of the usual suspects: cancer (24 percent), dementia and Alzheimer's (23 percent), vision loss (19 percent), heart disease (18 percent), and stroke (16 percent). They're the big, scary things that doctors have been warning us about from the moment we got our first cholesterol test.

But our number one health concern isn't one of those well-publicized conditions. It's just as scary, but something doctors don't really talk to us about: losing mobility. Thirty percent of those surveyed listed it among their top concerns, while an additional 14 percent listed falls and injuries. And losing mobility isn't a worry just for the oldest among us. It's the number one health concern among people ages fifty to fifty-nine. And that makes sense: Studies show that the speed at which we walk, known as our "gait speed," starts to decline in our mid-fifties, while our "fast gait speed"—essentially, how quickly we can go when we're really hustling—starts declining in our mid-forties.

Our fears are justified. Every eleven seconds, an older adult goes to an emergency department to treat an injury from a fall, according to the National Council on Aging, and every nineteen minutes, an older adult dies from a fall. It turns out that among older Americans, falls are the leading cause of both fatal and nonfatal injuries requiring hospitalization.

Mobility is a vulnerable asset, and its loss isn't always sudden. It starts with a creaky knee or a painful hip or an achy shoulder, and we learn to live with it, and adjust. But over time those accommodations to age pile up, until we're no longer engaging in the physical activities we once enjoyed, whether it's tennis or basketball or jogging or just gardening or taking long walks on the beach. It's often because we've gained weight in midlife, which takes a particular toll on the lower back, hips, and knees.

The lack of movement increases our risk of weight gain, which makes us even less mobile. Studies show that a body mass index over 30 increases an older person's risk of falling by as much as 78 percent.

Gaining back mobility, and preserving what you have, is one of the promises of the Whole Body Reset. By stopping age-related weight gain and bringing your weight back under control, you'll directly impact your mobility by reducing strain on your joints. By reducing inflammation, you'll significantly reduce your risk of joint pain. And by improving your overall health through both diet and exercise, you'll take back control of your gait, your balance . . . and your life.

A leaner, fitter body. A longer, healthier life. And a physical vitality that keeps us active and having fun well into our later years. This is what the Whole Body Reset can deliver for you. Your body wants and needs the healthy approach to nutrition and weight management that is the foundation of this program. Follow it—not religiously, but consciously to the best of your ability—and the rewards will be extraordinary.

Still . . . few of us go through life without bearing painful witness to the mental decline of someone we love, someone who may remain physically strong, but whose mind has been slowly stolen from them. That's why feeding the body is only part of our mission. The Whole Body Reset will also feed your mind, reducing your risk of age-related mental decline. In the next chapter, we'll explain how.

— ACTION STEP #6 —

When it comes to improving your health, eating better is move number one. But once you take charge of your diet, you're going to feel empowered to make other healthy changes as well. (Especially if you see the kind of improved energy levels our test panel reported!)

Research says that the best way to form a new, life-improving habit is to write down your goal, choose a simple action plan for getting there, and then set up a trigger that prompts you to perform the action at a certain place and time. So if your goal is to spend less time sitting, for example, you write down that goal, then add your plan—say, to move around more at work. Then add a trigger—for instance, "Every time I answer the phone, I'll stand up and walk around for five minutes." Try this simple pledge, or add your own particular life goal:

My goal is

_____

My plan is

_____

My trigger is

_____

I will

_____

Chapter 7

How the Whole Body Reset Can Help Keep Your Mind Sharp

The Untold Love Story of Your
Belly and Your Brain

When we think of cognitive decline, we tend to think of it as an inevitable result of aging, a genetic ticket that sooner or later gets punched.

But if we think of Alzheimer's disease and other forms of dementia as a natural byproduct of aging, we fail to see how much impact our choices today can have on our brains tomorrow. And one of the biggest life choices we make, several times a day, is the choice of what to eat. (How we exercise, too, impacts brain health; we get into that in Chapter 12, Your Whole Body Fitness Plan.)

"Understanding the interaction between nutrition and brain function is crucial as we age," Jean Woo, a member of the Global Council on Brain Health, told me. Woo is the Henry G. Leong Research Professor of Gerontology and Geriatrics and director of the Centre for Nutritional Studies at the Chinese University of Hong Kong.

Eating for a Healthy Brain

Nearly every single one of us has a story about a loved one lost to dementia. Let me tell you about one particular woman, the mother of a colleague of mine.

She was one of those people who was an indomitable force of nature, and she remained so well into her later years. Long after retirement, she held season's tickets to theater, ushered at the symphony, raised money for local candidates. She was active, engaged, involved—all the hallmarks of a stimulating, brain-healthy lifestyle.

But eating well was never a priority for her. She'd sip black coffee for breakfast, maybe eat a light lunch, and like many of us, consume most of her calories and protein at dinner—never skimping on dessert. Nighttime, you'd find her with a massive dish of ice cream—chocolate ripple, rocky road, moose tracks, anything chocolate—catching up on her magazines, mail, and email. She kept her mind active and social network wide, but her body grew larger, and her blood pressure and cholesterol levels responded accordingly.

In her seventies, she complained to her doctors that she was getting lost driving places she'd been going to for forty years; she couldn't remember if she'd taken her pills that morning. Neurologists ran tests, but her recall of the year and the president was excellent, and she could count backwards from one hundred by sevens faster than her daughter could. Doctors asked if she was getting enough sleep and mental stimulation, but never asked about her diet—despite her obvious weight problem. In her early eighties, doctors diagnosed mild cognitive disorder. They prescribed medications to slow the progression of brain decline but again, no questions about her diet. Ditto when, two years later, the diagnosis was dementia.

Those of us who have lost loved ones to dementia—and who, quite reasonably, worry about the same fate—understand how painful the

Brain Foods

Eat regularly

- Fresh vegetables (in particular, leafy greens such as spinach, chard, kale, arugula, collard greens, mustard greens, romaine lettuce, Swiss chard, turnip greens)
- Whole berries (not juice)
- Fish and seafood
- Healthy fats (e.g., extra-virgin olive oil, avocados, whole eggs)
- Nuts and seeds

Include

- Beans and other legumes
- Whole fruits (in addition to berries)
- Low-sugar, low-fat dairy (e.g., plain yogurt, cottage cheese)
- Poultry
- Whole grains

Limit

- Fried food
- Pastries, sugary foods
- Processed foods
- Red meat (e.g., beef, lamb, pork, buffalo, duck)
- Red meat products (e.g., bacon)
- Whole-fat dairy high in saturated fat, such as cheese and butter*
- Salt

Source: Global Council on Brain Health convened by AARP

* While the Global Council on Brain Health recommends only low-fat dairy for brain health, other studies have suggested full-fat products may have other benefits.

loss of brainpower can be, both to the sufferer and to those around them. That's one reason why, over the past several years, the world has focused more and more attention on understanding the brain, how it ages, and what we can do to slow its decline. And diet, experts have concluded, is one of the most powerful drivers of brain health.

The Global Council on Brain Health, an international collaborative of scientists and health experts convened by AARP, found that among people fifty and older, three-quarters of those who said they ate well five to seven times a week reported their brain health/mental sharpness as "excellent" or "very good." Of those who said they rarely or never ate healthfully, only 38 percent reported their brain health as high.

And here's the best news: It's never too late to start eating a healthy diet. "Improvements in your diet can help your brain health and lower your risks of cognitive decline whenever you decide to start," says Sarah Lenz Lock, the executive director of the Global Council on Brain Health.

Worried About Your Memory?

When you lose your car keys, do you worry that you're losing your mind? Three-quarters of adults aged forty and over are concerned about their brain health declining in the future, according to an AARP survey, and about one in three say they've noticed that their ability to remember things has decreased over the past five years. *Keep Sharp: Build a Better Brain at Any Age,* an AARP-supported book by Sanjay Gupta, MD, based in part on the work of AARP's Global Council on Brain Health, offers simple solutions for brain health. For a brain assessment and challenges, visit StayingSharp.org.

So, what's a "healthy" diet, in terms of your brain?

The Council has found that what's good for the heart is good for the brain. Not surprising, then, that the Mediterranean and DASH diets—long proven to improve heart health—look a lot like what you'll find in the pages of this book.

So start now. Here's how the Whole Body Reset can help you stay sharp for decades to come, reduce your risk of age-related brain diseases, and stave off mood swings and depression.

A Healthy Brain Needs Plenty of Fruits and Vegetables

One of the most significant effects of a plant-rich diet is its ability to feed the microbiome—the trillions of microscopic bacteria, fungi, and viruses that live in your gut and help with everything from digesting food to regulating the immune system. The microbiome also has a profound influence on the central nervous system. Dysregulated microbiomes have been linked to Alzheimer's, Parkinson's, depression, and other brain diseases.

"The gut influences the brain through two different pathways," Jean Woo told me. "One is through inflammation and a leaky gut, in which toxins leak from the gut and find a way to the brain." Inflammation is believed to play a crucial role in the development of dementia and other age-related brain diseases. The chemicals produced by the microbiome in the gut also stimulate the vagus nerve, which directly connects the brain and the digestive system and may also play a role in influencing our mood, our levels of inflammation, and our stress levels, among other crucial mind/body issues. A study by Woo and other researchers found that a higher intake of fruits and vegetables was tied to a reduced risk of age-related cognitive decline.

A brain-healthy diet means a wide array of plant foods, with a particular emphasis on leafy greens, which are rich in the brain-boosting nutrient folate, as well as vitamin K, lutein, and beta carotene, all of which have been linked to slowing cognitive decline. Nutrition researcher Katherine Tucker emphasizes the importance of getting not just a lot of plants, but a wide variety of plants, into your daily regimen for physical and brain health: "To keep down your inflammation and your oxidative stress, which are the two major things that damage your muscles and organs and contribute to development of chronic disease, you want to have not only the vitamins and minerals but also the phytochemicals and fiber that are found in fruits and vegetables and whole grains as well."

For that reason, it's plants, plants, plants, not pills, pills, pills. You can buy folate in pill form (as folic acid), but Tucker says research simply doesn't show that the pill form is effective. "Almost all the evidence shows that when you take things out of the food matrix and you put a single ingredient into a pill, it doesn't have the same effect," she says. For example, "We thought vitamin E was a major antioxidant, so in the 1990s everybody started taking vitamin E, and it turns out that it does not work." Many people continue to take vitamin E today, despite the fact that the Global Council on Brain Health has found that vitamin E in supplement form is not effective for brain health.

Get your nutrients from food, especially a variety of plant foods, and you reap all of the brain benefits. For brain health, the Whole Body Reset has you covered. You can't go wrong having at least one mixed salad a day, topped with a protein source or served alongside a protein-rich meal. Strive for 1½ to 2½ cups of vegetables a day, of all different colors, and two to four servings of fruit each day as well.

Which fruits? As with vegetables, variety is your best approach, although research seems to suggest that berries have a special place in the brain health pantheon. Scores of studies on animals have shown that strawberries, blackberries, blueberries, black currants, and mulberries all reduce inflammation in the nervous system.

A Healthy Brain Needs Less Sugar

Fruit punch could shrink your brain.

No, this is not a frantic Facebook message from your overly anxious Aunt Mary. This is actual scientific research: Regularly consuming sugary drinks leads to spiking blood sugar and an exaggerated insulin response, which can trigger chronic inflammation in the brain, making it vulnerable to Alzheimer's. A 2017 study linked high sugary beverage consumption to lower total brain volume, hippocampal volume, and poorer episodic memory.

But "sugary drinks" doesn't just mean the obvious culprits, like sodas and sweet teas. That 2017 study also looked at fruit punch and other fruit drinks,[1] and found them to be just as culpable. Be super careful of sugar hidden in "healthy" beverages such as juices and smoothies, sports drinks, and energy drinks, as well as specialty coffees. Some energy drinks can pack up to 60 grams of sugar in a 16-ounce can, while a 16-ounce vanilla latte may contain 35 grams. Frozen coffee drinks? Some pack more than 180 grams of sugar! That's more than you'd get if you ate a whole dozen apple cider donuts.

Now consider that one study of people with diabetes found that both memory and cognitive function decline faster with rising blood glucose levels.

The American Heart Association recommends that men consume no more than 150 calories (about 37.5 grams) of added sugar per day, and that women should limit their intake to no more than 100 calories (25 grams).[2] And yet one smoothie chain offers a "Fitness Blend" smoothie with 128 grams of sugar in it. That's 512 calories of pure sugary not-so-goodness.

Sugar in drinks damages the brain in the same way[3] that sugary food damages the body: by, among other things, raising your levels of inflammation.[4] And the Whole Body Reset reduces your sugar intake in two ways: first, by cutting calorie-laden drinks from your daily menu; and second, by filling you up with high-fiber, high-protein, high-nutrition foods that will tamp down hunger and sweet cravings, and keep you safe from sugar.

Boost Your Mood with the Whole Body Reset

Most of what's thought of as comfort food—macaroni and cheese, mashed potatoes and gravy, grilled cheese sandwiches, and French fries—ought to be called discomfort food, especially if it's processed or fried in oil derived from corn or soy. Those oils are high in omega-6 fatty acids, a type of fat linked to inflammation and depression. In older adults, high levels of omega-6 fatty acids were associated with a higher rate of depression, according to a study in *Psychosomatic Medicine*. So instead of grabbing something fatty and sad, reach for something lean and happy.

Leafy greens. Having low blood levels of magnesium and a low intake of magnesium from foods are both associated with an increased risk of depression. Fill up on magnesium-rich dark, leafy greens such as spinach, as well as pumpkin seeds, almonds, peanut butter, and legumes.

Protein in the morning. Protein may help synthesize serotonin, a brain hormone responsible for helping to lower anxiety and to boost mood.

Fatty fish. It's rich in the omega-3 fatty acids EPA and DHA, which have been shown to improve symptoms of moderate and major depression and to reduce anxiety significantly.

A Healthy Brain Needs Less Salt and More Potassium and Calcium

High blood pressure can damage small blood vessels in the brain, hindering our memory and our thinking ability. That's why controlling it is so important: In fact, researchers report that when people with high blood pressure take potassium-sparing diuretics or thiazide diuretics, their risk of developing Alzheimer's is significantly reduced.

And since we know that sodium can play an enormous role in elevating blood pressure, it's no surprise that health organizations continue to urge us to avoid the white stuff. In one study, a 50 percent reduction in salt cut the risk of a fatal stroke by 85 percent. The American Heart Association recommends no more than 1,500 milligrams of sodium a day (that's a little less than ¾ teaspoon of salt), while the *Dietary Guidelines* suggests no more than 2,300 milligrams (a full teaspoon).

Problem is, sticking to those guidelines is extremely difficult, especially when you're eating at a restaurant or getting takeout. Just about every chain hamburger or sub you can find weighs in at close to 1,000 milligrams of sodium (some hit twice that amount), and that's before the fries. Soups, sandwiches, burritos, and pizza are among the top sources of sodium in the American diet, according to the Centers for Disease Control, which pretty much wipes out most fast-food joints. And even making lunch at home is tough: A simple turkey sandwich with mustard, lettuce, and cheese can cost you more than 1,500 milligrams of sodium (690 milligrams from the turkey, and as much as an additional 300 milligrams from the two slices of bread). We give you lots of options that go light on salt while heavy on taste—see the recipes in Chapter 14. On the Whole Body Reset, you'll naturally cut your sodium level.

But honestly, controlling sodium intake is not always possible. You will go out to eat. You will eat bread and burgers and pizza. And you know we're not about deprivation. Fortunately, even as you watch your sodium intake, the Whole Body Reset gives you a number of weapons to lower blood pressure. Follow this program, and you'll take real steps toward lowering your blood pressure naturally by controlling your weight and exercising more. But just as important, you'll boost your intake of calcium and potassium, both of which—as we learned in the previous chapter—help to control blood pressure.

Meanwhile, it's important to see your doctor regularly and monitor your blood pressure. If you're prescribed blood pressure medicine, take it—the risks to your heart, and your brain, from uncontrolled blood pressure is simply too high to fool around with.

A Healthy Brain Needs More Fish and More Healthy Fats

Among people in olive-growing regions, the incidence of cognitive decline—along with heart disease, cancer, and type 2 diabetes—is very low.

"We've known for fifty or sixty years that the Mediterranean diet is beneficial for health, but olive oil is emerging as the most important ingredient," says Domenico Praticò, MD, director of the Alzheimer's Center at Temple University.

Take people in the Sicani Mountain region of Sicily, marked by rolling hills covered with olive trees. These mountainfolk eat a Mediterranean diet, high in fish, whole grains, and fruits and vegetables. But their community, and their daily diet, revolves around olive trees; they snack on olives and use the fruit's unprocessed oil (what we know as extra-virgin olive oil, or EVOO) to prepare dinner. As a result, their arteries are as supple as those of people ten years younger, researchers say. And that helps keep their brains younger, too, says Woo. "Brain health and heart health are both mediated by blood vessels, and what you eat determines whether those vessels will clog up or not. The same things that give rise to the clogging of the vessels in the heart may also give rise to clogging in the brain." But, she says, the brain is even more vulnerable to this process than the heart is. While both organs have the ability to grow new blood vessels that circumnavigate clogged arteries, the brain is less capable of utilizing this vascular superpower, because its network of blood vessels is more complex.

Healthy fats like EVOO can do more than just keep your blood vessels pristine. Researchers have recently discovered that compounds in the fat of this high-grade oil can flush out proteins that gum up the communication channels between brain cells, slowing disease progression. One particular compound that seems to drive this effect is an olive-derived polyphenol called oleocanthal. In animal studies at Auburn University, oleocanthal demonstrated an ability to rinse out amyloids, which form the plaques associated with Alzheimer's. In mice, EVOO can flush out tau, a protein that hinders language skills and memory in humans. Of course, there's a huge gap between promising animal studies and hard evidence that EVOO has the same effect on our human brains. But it's promising. And also, delicious.

Note that important acronym: EVOO. Extra-virgin olive oil. The difference between EVOO and your everyday olive oil is sort of like the difference between whole grain bread and processed white bread. EVOO is higher in polyphenols (those heart-healthy, brain-healthy nutrients); regular olive oil is processed and has much lower levels of these essential nutrients.

The very factors that make EVOO a brain-healthy fat—it's plant-based and the least processed—extend to other types of fat as well. Avocados, nuts, seeds, and peanuts are all brain healthy because

---

Progress, Not Perfection

With each meal, you have the power to make a healthy choice for your brain—even if your diet isn't exactly perfect. In a study of subjects following a brain-healthy diet, researchers found that those who followed the diet most closely (an average score of 9.6 points out of a possible 15) saw the biggest drop in their Alzheimer's risk. But those whose adherence was a little sketchy (scoring 7.5 points out of 15) still cut their risk by over a third.

---

they're loaded with monounsaturated fats, and so, too, are the oils derived from these plants. A study of more than fifteen thousand older women found that eating nuts five or more times a week correlated with a lower rate of cognitive decline compared to women who never ate nuts. (The study was partially funded by the California Walnuts Commission, but also by the highly respected National Institute on Aging.)

Omega-3 fatty acids are also among the good fats you should know about if you're concerned about shrinking brains. And really, who wouldn't be? Reduced brain volume that comes with age is correlated to increased incidence of Alzheimer's disease.

Research shows that omega-3s fight inflammation and support the structure of brain cells. A 2011 report in *Neurology* by researchers at Oregon Health & Science University found that study participants who had high blood levels of healthy fats, including omega-3s, low levels of trans fats, plus a variety of vitamins (including B, C, D, and E) had less brain shrinkage and scored better on cognitive tests than those who ate less-nutritious diets.

The bottom line is this: We have a considerable amount of influence on the direction of our short- and long-term brain health, and one of the most potent arrows in our quiver is diet. To stay sharp now and long into the future, you've come to the right place.

A Healthy Brain Needs More Fiber

Yes, you're getting older. And so is your microbiome, a collection of trillions of bacteria that live in and on your body, primarily in your gut. And the health of those bugs in your belly can have a big impact on your brain.

If you've ever felt your stomach tied up in knots when you sit in traffic or filled up with butterflies before giving a talk, you've experienced the powerful effects of the enteric nervous system, often called the "brain in your gut." This system is made up of the thousands of nerves that line the digestive tract and the same neurotransmitters, such as serotonin, that govern mood.

This intricate gut-brain connection sends electrical messages back and forth, signaling whether you're hungry, stressed, depressed, or feeling just fine. For example, Australian researchers found that students had lower levels of lactic acid bacteria, a good type of gut bacteria, during exam week, compared with less stressful times in the semester. On the other hand, your digestive tract also manufactures as much as 90 percent of the body's serotonin, the feel-good hormone that regulates mood.

To carry out these complicated tasks, the gut uses beneficial bacteria called probiotics. We get probiotics from certain foods, particularly fermented foods like yogurt and kimchi, that are rich in these types of bacteria. But we also nourish our existing probiotics by feeding them fiber, which helps them grow and flourish.

The Whole Body Reset is rich in whole grains, fruits, vegetables, and other fiber-rich foods that support the gut. But for an extra brain boost, invest in the following:

1. **Yogurt.** UCLA researchers gave a group of healthy women either probiotic-rich yogurt, a probiotic-free milk product, or neither. At the start of the study, the women had MRI scans of the brain measuring their reaction to pictures of people with angry or frightened faces. After four weeks, the MRI scans were repeated using the same pictures. Overall, the women who ate yogurt responded more calmly, while the other groups tended to show either the same response they had originally or a heightened response. Kefir (a yogurt-like beverage) is also rich in probiotics.

2. **Cold cooked potatoes.** Potatoes are high in the kind of starch the body digests quickly, causing blood pressure and insulin to surge and then dip. But cooking and then chilling the spuds alters their chemical makeup; they develop a specific type of starch that resists digestion in the small intestine. This resistant starch passes to the colon undigested and, once there, serves as a prebiotic to feed the healthy bacteria that live in the gut.

3. **Onions, leeks, and garlic.** This dynamic prebiotic trio, members of the allium family, is one of the best sources of a soluble fiber called oligofructose, a natural source of inulin. Studies show that inulin stimulates the growth of healthy bacteria, which forces out potentially harmful bugs trying to gain a toehold. In addition, some research suggests that alliums may help the body resist infection, boost brain performance, help protect the heart, and control cholesterol.

4. **Refrigerated sauerkraut.** This tangy probiotic and its cousins kimchi and sour pickles are a great way to restore healthy gut bacteria after a course of antibiotics. They contain live bacteria that can help repopulate the gut as well as bacteria and enzymes that help the body absorb some nutrients more readily. Look for fermented vegetables that are refrigerated, not shelf-stable

canned or bottled products, which have been preserved using vinegar—a process that kills off most of the healthy bacteria. Kombucha tea is another source of healthy gut bacteria.

A Healthy Brain Needs Healthy Muscles, Too

What do you think of when you hear the word "muscles"?

- Sylvester Stallone, Arnold Schwarzenegger, and other strangely sinuous septuagenarians
- Strains, sprains, and pains
- A bucket of steamy black shellfish
- A proven key to extending your mental wellness far into the future

The Whole Body Reset is focused on helping you preserve muscle as you grow older, and it's not just because we want you to look good in a T-shirt. In a study of 3,000 adults ages fifty-four to eighty-nine, researchers found that having a strong grip was inversely related to symptoms of depression; the stronger you are, the less likely you are to be clinically depressed.

But the power of muscle can go beyond just our mood. Studies also show that having strong muscles may help protect us against the loss of cognitive function as we age. One study looked at 970 people living in senior communities who had no evidence of cognitive decline. Researchers put the subjects through a series of strength tests, measuring their upper and lower extremities. Adjusting for variables like sex and age, the researchers ranked participants' strength on a scale of -1.6 (weakest) to 3.3 (strongest). Over the next 3.6 years, 15 percent of the subjects developed Alzheimer's. But their risk was largely determined by where they fell on the strength scale:

For every 1 point increase in muscle strength, a subject's risk of Alzheimer's dropped by 43 percent![5]

In another study of adults (average age: sixty-three) researchers used PET and CT scans to determine how much lean muscle subjects had. They found that increased muscle mass was linked to a lower risk of Alzheimer's.[6]

And it's not just your risk of future decline that's at stake. One study found that having low muscle mass was an indicator of low executive function—meaning, the ability to focus, stay organized, and generally run your life. It's ironic, when you consider the stereotype of "dumb jocks," to see how clearly retaining muscle mass is linked to retaining smarts.

— ACTION STEP #7 —

More and more research is finding that healthy fats—such as monounsaturated fats from olives, avocados, and nuts, as well as omega-3 fatty acids from fish, soy, walnuts, and seeds—play a crucial role in warding off cognitive decline. Pick five ways you can incorporate healthy fats into your diet to help keep your brain functioning at its very best. (For example, use olive oil in place of corn oil, or add walnuts to your salad, or have a tuna instead of a turkey sandwich.)

1 _____

2 _____

3 _____

4 _____

5 _____

Chapter 8

Your Magic Supermarket Label Decoder

How to Find the Best
Foods for Your Body

There's a very simple mantra that diet experts like to repeat: "Eat whole foods." They're talking about foods that have only one ingredient: Apples. Chicken. Broccoli. Brown rice. Almonds. That sort of thing. And if you want to reset your whole body, then for sure, you want to eat more whole foods.

But that's not how the real world operates. Sometimes, we need to buy something that's prepared and then packaged in a box, bag, or can, and there is simply no such thing as a one-ingredient pasta sauce, or salad dressing, or loaf of bread. But there are simple ways to select the most nutritious packaged foods on the market, whether we're buying a necessity or an indulgence. So join us on a trip through the grocery store and discover how easy it is to upgrade your shopping cart.

But . . . before we leave, you'll want to make a list of all that you need to buy—and do your best to actually stick to the list. As you'll see below, supermarkets are brilliant when it comes to getting you to buy stuff you didn't intend to buy. And if you make a smart list, you're going to come away with a lot of nutritious food; studies show that list-makers are more prone to make healthy choices. Planning, as the old generals used to say, is everything.

Supermarket Treasure Map

Ever make a shopping list, then discover that what's in your cart at checkout is about twice what you intended to buy? Or pop into the supermarket for milk and bread and come out with a box of weird chocolate doohickies?

Supermarkets are data-driven Venus flytraps, designed to lure us in and then envelop us in an inescapable embrace of consumerism. Their very layouts are cleverly designed to play with our minds.

Consider:

The produce is always right by the front door. Why? Because when you see it, you're immediately given a boost of confidence in your health-focused shopping plan. In fact, you feel so good about those fruits and vegetables that you don't mind piling a few extra boxes of snacks in your cart as you cruise the aisles.

The milk and eggs are always at the back. Don't supermarkets realize that we all need to purchase dairy items on pretty much every trip? They do, which is why they want us to have to traverse a maze of brightly colored snackables before we find what we came for, all the better to tempt us with. You'll also find the meat and seafood along the walls.

The middle of the store is a big waist-land. The perimeter of the store is where the most nutritious foods are found, while the center aisles—where it's easy to get lost and confused—contain most of the refined foods. Here's where a shopping list can really save you: When you dive into the middle passages, try to stick to what you're there to buy, and read labels carefully.

choices, on the other hand, have higher totals of protein and fiber than sugar.

For example, consider breakfast cereals. Here are some of the healthy breakfast cereals with more protein + fiber totals than sugar:

Fiber One Honey Clusters Lightly Sweetened Flakes

Protein 4 g + Fiber 10 g = 14 g

Sugars 9 g

Kellogg's All-Bran, Original

Protein 4 g + Fiber 10 g = 14 g

Sugars 6 g

Cheerios

Protein 5 g + Fiber 4 g = 9 g

Sugars 2 g

Unfortunately, most cereals on the market don't meet this standard. And be careful even within brands. For example, compare regular Cheerios with Honey Nut Cheerios:

Cheerios, Honey Nut

Protein 3 g + Fiber 3 g = 6 g

Sugars 12 g

A lot of products are naturally loaded with protein and fiber, and you'd probably assume they'd fit within this formula. But never underestimate food manufacturers' ability to take something good, and make it not as good. For example, baked beans. How could beans—rich with protein and fiber—not be a smart choice? Let's take a look.

Bush's Steakhouse Recipe Grillin' Beans

Protein 7 g + Fiber 5 g = 12 g

Sugars 19 g

Heinz Kentucky Style Bourbon and Molasses BBQ Baked Beans

Protein 7 g + Fiber 5 g = 12 g

Sugars 18 g

Hanover Country Style Baked Beans

Protein 7 g + Fiber 6 g = 13 g

Sugars 14 g

Let's note here that each of these manufacturers also makes plenty of healthier bean products. For example:

Hanover Great Northern Beans

Protein 7 g + Fiber 7 g = 14 g

Sugars 0 g

The point is, get used to reading the labels and looking at these three data points. It will help guide you when choosing between products that look similar.

For example, let's say you're shopping for a carb to accompany your morning eggs. Here are three sets of products that look almost identical—but they're not.

Let's start with tortillas:

Mission Garden Spinach Herb Wraps

Protein 6 g + Fiber 1 g = 7 g

Sugars 1 g

Mission Carb Balance Spinach Wraps

Protein 6 g + Fiber 15 g = 21 g

Sugars 0 g

Both products will wrap your huevos rancheros nicely, but the Carb Balance version crushes it with far more fiber and a little less sugar.

What about just some sliced bread for toast?

Arnold Country Style Oatmeal Bread (2 slices)

Protein 10 g + Fiber 2 g = 12 g

Sugars 6 g

Arnold Whole Grains 12 Grain Bread (2 slices)

Protein 10 g + Fiber 6 g = 16 g

Sugars 4 g

Both seem worthy of a visit to your toaster, but the 12-grain bread has more protein, more fiber, and less sugar. Why wouldn't you make this choice?

Rather have an English muffin? Let's check these out:

Thomas's Cinnamon Raisin English Muffins

Protein 4 g + Fiber 2 g = 6 g

Sugars 8 g

Thomas's Whole Wheat English Muffins

Protein 5 g + Fiber 3 g = 8 g

Sugars 1 g

Both muffins have similar protein and fiber counts, but the cinnamon raisin has eight times the sugar!

By applying this mathematical formula, you may even find healthy choices in unexpected places. For example, can you imagine a healthy candy bar? Here are three:

Green & Black's Organic Dark Chocolate Bar, 85% Cacao (10 squares)

Protein 3 g + Fiber 4 g = 7 g

Sugars 4 g

What Does This Word Mean?

If you want to evaluate any given food product, it helps to ignore all meaningless words and marketing lingo. For example:

- **Multigrain:** Just means there's a lot of different types of carbs. But it doesn't mean they're whole grain or healthy.
- **Diet:** Reduced-calorie products often contain fewer nutrients and more fillers. Avoid products with "diet" labels and choose based on what you see on the nutrition panels.
- **Premium:** At best this means "more expensive."
- **Natural:** So's bird poop. "Natural" is meaningless as a marketing term, with no definition established by the U.S. government.
- **Artisanal:** Seems to imply there's a secret cache of Italian grandmothers being held captive in the factory. Beyond that, it's pretty vague.
- **Homemade:** This is only true if the Italian grandmothers are forced to live in the same factory where they work. That's just cruel!

On the other hand, some words do have meaning, signaling that you're making a healthier choice. For example:

Lindt Excellence 85% Dark Chocolate Bar (4 squares)

Protein 5 g + Fiber 6 g = 11 g

Sugars 5 g

Ghirardelli 86% Cacao Midnight Reverie Bar (2½ squares)

Protein 2 g + Fiber 4 g = 6 g

Sugars 3 g

- **Low Sodium:** This is a government-regulated term that means the product has less than 140 milligrams of sodium per serving. "Reduced sodium," on the other hand, means only that the product has at least 25 percent less than the original product— meaning it could still be loaded with the salty stuff.
- **Low-fat:** This means 3 grams or less of fat per serving. But again, "reduced fat" means that the product has at least 25 percent less fat than the original product, and these products tend to be higher in sugar.
- **Lite or Light:** The FDA lets manufacturers use these terms if the food has less fat, calories, or sodium than similar foods. But like "low-fat," beware of added sugars to compensate.
- **100% whole grains or 100% whole wheat:** Look for the Whole Grain Stamp, which indicates the percentage of carbs that are whole grain. A 100% Stamp means it's all whole grain, with at least 16 grams per labeled serving. A 50%+ Stamp means at least half is whole grain, with at least 8 grams per labeled serving. A Basic Stamp says the product contains at least 8 grams of whole grain.

These are intensely dark chocolate, and not to everyone's taste. But they show how the most unexpected foods really do qualify as "health" foods, if you look at them through this simple mathematical lens.

This doesn't mean all foods that have more fiber and protein than sugar are good for you. You could live within this guideline on a diet of salted chips and bacon. But when you're choosing between products, or trying to decide if a packaged food is the best choice, doing this quick calculation can serve as a foundation.

Understanding Added Sugars

One more stop before we move out of those middle aisles. Starting in 2020, the USDA required all packaged foods to reflect not just total sugars, but "added sugars." Added sugar refers to what's not normally found in the food itself, but rather added by the manufacturer. A glass of milk contains a certain amount of naturally occurring sugar (known as lactose); stir in some chocolate mix, and you've got added sugars.

This requirement is a great step forward for those who are looking to fully understand how nutritious (or not) our food is. Many of our most nutritious foods—particularly fruit and dairy—come with a decent amount of natural sugar, which is nature's way of encouraging us to eat them. The term "added sugars" refers to when manufacturers "improve" our food by adding one of many different types of sweetener—sweeteners with little to no nutritional value. Here's just a sampling of added sugars you might find snuck into your favorite foods:

Sweet Nothings

Agave nectar	Dextrose	Maple syrup
Anhydrous dextrose	Evaporated cane juice	Molasses
Beet sugar	Fructose	Pancake syrup
Brown rice syrup	Fruit juice concentrates	Powdered sugar
Brown sugar	Fruit nectars	Raw sugar
Cane crystals	Glucose	Rice syrup
Coconut palm sugar	High fructose corn syrup	Sucrose
Confectioner's sugar	Honey	Sugar
Corn sweetener	Invert sugar	Sugar cane syrup
Corn syrup	Lactose	Table sugar
Corn syrup solids	Maltose	Turbinado
Crystalline fructose	Malt syrup	White granulated sugar

Let's see how "added sugars" help change the nature of what would normally be a healthy food choice. Start with something simple:

Chobani Low-Fat Plain Greek Yogurt (¾ cup serving)

Calories 130

Total Sugars 4 g

Added Sugars 0 g

Fiber 0 g

Protein 17 g

This is a pretty unadulterated food; just low-fat yogurt, nothing added. And, as you see, it has 4 grams of naturally occurring sugar from the milk itself.

Now what happens when the manufacturer adds sugar?

Chobani 2% Greek Yogurt, Mango (⅔ cup serving)

Calories 130

Total Sugars 14 g

Added Sugars 9 g

Fiber 0 g

Protein 11 g

Whoa, what just happened? Well, after yogurt and mango, the third ingredient on the nutrition label is "cane sugar." And because of that, you've crossed the Rubicon into less-healthy territory.

On the other hand, if you had cut up ⅓ cup of mango and added it to the plain yogurt, you would have added 8 grams of natural sugars and a gram of fiber. So your protein + fiber content would still outweigh your sugar content.

Chobani Low-Fat Plain Greek Yogurt plus ⅓ cup mango

Calories 165

Dairy Sugars 4 g + Mango Sugars 8 g = Total Sugars 12 g

Added Sugars 0 g

Fiber 1 g

Protein 17 g

The Dairy Case

If you're health-conscious, you may instinctively reach for low-fat versions of your favorite dairy products. You may even sometimes wrestle with yourself or members of your family over how low you can go: Is coffee still palatable with skim milk? Does fat-free plain yogurt still taste good? Or should you go with 1 percent or 2 percent versions, as a compromise?

Stop having these arguments. Because the truth is, low-fat versions of dairy products, besides cutting calories, may not offer any other real benefits: One study, for example, found that those who ate three servings of dairy had lower risks of heart disease and stroke than those who ate one serving[1]—regardless of whether they ate whole-fat or reduced-fat versions. The fact is that that there are many conflicting studies about the impact of dairy fat on heart health. What we do know is that calcium and vitamin D are hard to get anywhere else, and crucial for your overall health, regardless of what form of dairy you choose.

That doesn't mean that you should be drinking cream and melted butter: A cup of whole milk has 8 grams of fat, while a cup of butter has 184 grams. And it doesn't mean ice cream is now a health food— frozen dairy desserts are usually loaded with unhealthy added sugars, regardless of fat content. But it does mean that if you like whole-fat dairy, feel free to skip the skim—especially if the extra fat inspires you to have cottage cheese, Greek yogurt, a slice of cheese, or a cup of milk more often.

Of course, plenty of people can't stomach milk, or other lactose-containing dairy foods. If that's you, don't be fooled into thinking that all dairy alternatives are the same. Most are very low in protein,

Milky Waze
Per 1 Cup (unsweetened)

	CALORIES	PROTEIN	FAT	CALCIUM
Skim milk	101	10 g	0 g	300 mg
Whole milk	149	8 g	8 g	300 mg
Pea milk	70	8 g	4.5 g	451 mg
Soy milk	105	6 g	3.5 g	300 mg
Oat milk	101	4 g	1.5 g	19 mg
Flax hemp milk	46	2 g	3 g	29 mg
Almond milk	90	1 g	2.5 g	451 mg
Coconut milk	76	0.5 g	5 g	459 mg

so they aren't really "substitutes" at all. If you choose to go with a non-dairy alternative, opt for soy milk or a pea protein blend, both of which deliver about ¾ the protein of regular milk; be sure to pick a brand that is fortified with calcium and, ideally, vitamin D as well.

Meat, Poultry, and Seafood

The very idea of meat on the plate stands for prosperity; like apple pie, Superman, and Chevy convertibles, meat on the dinner plate is straight-up Americana.

But too much meat isn't a good thing. When you're ordering that 22-ounce steak at the popular chain restaurant, you're actually getting more than four times the protein that your body needs—and can use. (Remember, we can process only about 30 to 40 grams of protein at a time.) All that money, all those calories . . . for naught. That's one reason why cooking meat at home is not only a less expensive option, but a healthier one as well.

Red Meat

The USDA requires most commercially sold red meat to be labeled as either prime, choice, or select. All of those sound pretty good, but what do they mean? The rankings have to do with how much fat, or marbling, is in the meat itself. But regardless of the grade of meat, the protein, vitamin, and mineral contents are similar.

- **Prime:** Abundant marbling, which means the meat is deeply flavorful and juicy, but also higher in fat than other grades.

- **Choice:** Less marbling than prime, but still relatively well-flecked with fat.

- **Select:** Leaner than higher grades, still tender, but lower in fat. Usually cuts with "round," "chuck," or "loin" in their name.

- **Extra Lean:** Least amount of fat.

Lean into Meat

Keywords that indicate a lower-fat cut:

Beef: eye of round, top round, sirloin, top loin, tenderloin

Pork: tenderloin, top loin, sirloin, loin chop, rib chop

Lamb: leg of lamb, arm, loin

So if flavor is your primary focus and cost isn't an issue, it may make sense to stick with one of the higher grades. But if you want meat that's leaner and less expensive, Select might be the way to go—especially if you're dressing it up with marinades or mixing it into another dish. Game meats such as bison or venison are very lean and rich in zinc and iron. Depending on where you are in the country, you may find game meat in the market or you may have to order online. You do not have to hunt them to eat them.

And now, more than ever, you can find meat substitutes loaded with protein.

Burger Nutrition Comparison

Nutrition information serving size	Ground beef 80% lean, 20% fat (100 grams)	Beyond Burger (113 grams)	Impossible Burger (113 grams)	Morning Star Black Bean (67 grams)	Boca Burger (71 grams)
Calories	270 calories	290 calories	240 calories	110 calories	100 calories
Saturated Fat	6.7g	5g	8g	0.5g	1g
Protein	26g	20g	19g	9g	13g
Sodium	75mg	450mg	370mg	320mg	350mg

Poultry

Chicken is the inexpensive go-to for lean meat. But unlike red meat, which offers so many different grades and cuts, your chicken choice is pretty much limited: breast or legs?

Of course, food marketers hate clarity. Hence, you'll find other terms on packages of chicken, many of which will lead you to believe that your dinner was recently running wild on verdant acres of natural farmland. The truth is a little less idyllic. Here's how to decode a package of chicken:

Air-chilled: It's standard for slaughtered chickens, during processing, to be dunked in frigid bath water to keep bacteria at a minimum. When immersed in their cold-water baths, poultry can absorb up to 12 percent of their weight in water, which dilutes flavor and is, yes, kinda icky. (Plus, that means 12 percent of your money is going to water, not chicken.) "Air-chilled" means the processor skipped this step, and instead chilled the chicken in a refrigerator unit. This cools the chicken more slowly, which may render the meat more tender and less water-saturated. (Look also for the term "no retained water.")

Free-range: Technically, a "free-range" bird must have access to the outdoors, but the USDA does not strictly define "outdoors." So the "range" may have just been a puny hole in the coop from which the chicken could stick out its head.

Organic: A truly organic chicken was raised on organic feed and had access to pasture. Look for the USDA Organic seal, which guarantees you're getting what's advertised.

Seafood

On one hand, you know that seafood delivers lean protein, and that many types of seafood contain a healthy serving of omega-3 fatty acids, which have been linked to improved brain and cardiovascular health. On the other hand, you've probably heard plenty of scary stories about mercury and other contaminants in fish, enough that you're wondering whether "meat without feet" really is a healthy alternative. The fact is, most commercial seafood is relatively low in contaminants, and safe enough to eat on a weekly basis, with only a handful that should give you real pause.

As you're going down the seafood aisle, whether fresh or frozen, consider the following list, adapted from the Berkeley Wellness newsletter, ranking seafood according to its omega-3 content. Those highlighted in **bold** are very low in contaminants and can be eaten several times a week. The others have moderate levels, but are still safe to eat even on a weekly basis.

More than 1,500 milligrams omega-3:
> **herring, wild (Atlantic and Pacific); salmon, farmed (Atlantic); salmon, wild (king); mackerel, wild (Pacific and jack)**

1,000 to 1,500 milligrams omega-3:
> **salmon, canned (pink, sockeye, and chum); mackerel, canned (jack); mackerel, wild (Atlantic);** mackerel, wild (Atlantic and Spanish); tuna, wild (bluefin)

500 to 1,000 milligrams omega-3:
> **salmon, wild (sockeye, coho, chum, and pink); sardines, canned; tuna, canned (white albacore);** swordfish, wild; **trout, farmed (rainbow); oysters, wild and farmed**; mussels, wild and farmed

200 to 500 milligrams omega-3:
> **tuna, canned (light); tuna, wild (skipjack); pollock, wild (Alaskan);** rockfish, wild (Pacific); **clams, wild and farmed; crab, wild (king, Dungeness, and snow); lobster, wild (spiny);** snapper, wild; grouper, wild; **flounder/sole, wild;** halibut, wild (Pacific and Atlantic); ocean perch, wild; **squid, wild (fried);** fish sticks (breaded)

How to Buy a Tasty, Brain-Healthy Oil

Extra-virgin olive oil has been shown to lower cholesterol levels, blood pressure, and the risk of Alzheimer's, stroke, and death from heart disease. Oleocanthal, the polyphenol in the oil, has also been shown to rinse out Alzheimer's plaques in mice. That's a major reason extra-virgin is the go-to olive oil for the Whole Body Reset.

Here's how to find the right product for you:

1. **Look for the "extra-virgin."** That distinction means the oil is free of flavor defects and contains the highest concentration of disease-fighting polyphenols.

2. **Pick a dark bottle.** Olives are fruit, and olive oil is a fruit juice. As with any juice, exposure to light can destroy those polyphenols. Dark glass or tins offer much better protection for the precious nutrients. For further protection, store the oil in a cool, dark place.

3. **Check the bottle date.** To find the freshest oil, look for the best-before date, which is usually eighteen to twenty-four months from when the oil was bottled. And don't buy bigger bottles than you'll need, since once you open the bottle and expose the oil to oxygen, it begins to degrade.

4. **Give it a swig.** The more potent an oil's flavor, the more powerful its protective effects. If you feel a slight burn in the back of your throat, it means the oil has high levels of oleocanthal.

Less than 200 milligrams omega-3:
**scallops, wild; shrimp, wild and farmed; lobster, wild
(northern); crab, wild (blue); cod, wild; haddock, wild; tilapia,
farmed; catfish, farmed;** mahimahi, wild; tuna, wild (yellowfin);
orange roughy, wild; surimi product (imitation crab)

*Pregnant women, women who might become pregnant, and young
children should avoid:*
Bigeye tuna, king mackerel, marlin, orange roughy, shark,
swordfish, tilefish (from the Gulf of Mexico)

Source: seafoodhealthfacts.org/ and Berkeley Wellness.

You may have read about issues of overfishing in our oceans, and
how poor fishing practices threaten the health of our oceans. Check
out seafoodwatch.org/recommendations to find sustainable seafood
choices.

— ACTION STEP #8 —

Even if you love food, and you love shopping, chances are you don't
love food shopping. Weird, right? And yet we spend more time
doing it now than ever before—the average food shopper spends
about forty-six minutes each day they shop, up 6 percent from a
decade earlier, according to the USDA. Let's make your next grocery shopping—whether it's at the supermarket, the big box store,
or simply online—both easier and healthier.

List three supermarket products you commonly buy, and then
play a little like Nancy Drew: Identify product swaps you can make
to increase the amount of nutrients you're eating while enjoying the
same kind of food. For example, instead of your usual brand-name
pasta, maybe you can try a whole wheat or "pulse" pasta version
(meaning a type of high-protein pasta made from chickpeas, lentils,

or other legume) to up your whole grain intake. Or find a similar packaged product that has less sugar, more fiber, or more protein— or all of the above!

Instead of _____ ,

eat _____

Instead of _____ ,

eat _____

Instead of _____ ,

eat _____

The Whole Body Reset Shopping List—and Some "Health Foods" That Are NOT on Your List!

Never say never. The occasional candy bar, slice of bacon, or bowl of cereal with a cartoon on the box won't hurt you. But with this shopping list, filled with tasty foods, you'll feel truly satisfied, strengthen your body, and lose weight or prevent age-related weight gain.

Produce Section

Fill your cart with all sorts of colorful produce—try some you've never tasted! Here are some suggestions. (Fresh, frozen, and canned are all fine, so long as they don't have added sugars.)

Fruits

GOOD FOR YOUR WHOLE BODY

Apples	Melon
Avocados	Nectarines
Bananas	Oranges
Berries	Papaya
Cherries	Peaches
Dried fruit (such as raisins, apricots, figs)	Pears
Grapefruit	Pineapple
Kiwi	Plums
Mango	Star fruit

NOT GOOD FOR YOUR WHOLE BODY

Fruit products such as roll-ups or jams

Canned fruit in syrup

Sugar-added dried fruit such as Craisins

Vegetables

GOOD FOR YOUR WHOLE BODY

Artichoke

Asparagus

Beets

Boy choy

Broccoli

Broccoli rabe

Brussels sprouts

Cabbage

Carrots

Cauliflower

Celery

Eggplant

Fennel

Herbs (such as basil and parsley)

Leafy greens (such as arugula, collard, kale, romaine, spinach, Swiss chard)

Leeks

Onion (yellow, white, red)

Peas

Peppers

Potatoes (sweet and white)

Snap peas

Squash

Turnips

Dairy Section *(Any fat content is fine.)*

GOOD FOR YOUR WHOLE BODY

Cottage cheese

Eggs

Greek yogurt, plain, or yogurts that have more protein than sugar

Hard and soft cheeses

Kefir, fortified

Ricotta cheese

NOT GOOD FOR YOUR WHOLE BODY

Cottage cheese and fruit cups with added sugar

Eggs in milk cartons

Meat and Poultry Aisle *(Choose lean cuts of meat.)*

GOOD FOR YOUR WHOLE BODY

Burgers	Pork
Chicken	Turkey
Lamb	Venison

NOT GOOD FOR YOUR WHOLE BODY

Cured or processed meats

Nuggets and other breaded chicken

Seafood *(Focus on omega-3 rich fish, fresh, frozen, and canned.)*

GOOD FOR YOUR WHOLE BODY

Herring	Salmon
Mackerel	Trout
Mussels	Tuna
Oysters	

NOT GOOD FOR YOUR WHOLE BODY

Fish low in omega-3s (catfish, imitation crab, tilapia)

Breaded fish sticks

Plant- and Whey-Based Protein *(These items are in different places in different stores, so ask your grocer if you can't find them.)*

GOOD FOR YOUR WHOLE BODY

Edamame (usually with frozen foods)

Nut and seed butter, 100%

Nuts (almonds, cashews, pistachios, walnuts)
Plant-based high-protein burger substitutes (usually with
    frozen foods or meats)
Seeds (chia, flax, hemp, pumpkin, and sunflower seeds)
Seitan
Soy or pea milk
Tempeh
Tofu

NOT GOOD FOR YOUR WHOLE BODY
Candied nuts
Low-protein burger substitutes
Nut butters with added sugars
Oat, almond, coconut, or other low-protein milks

Fats
GOOD FOR YOUR WHOLE BODY
Extra-virgin olive oil
Nut and seed oils
Olive oil cooking spray
Olives, green or black

NOT GOOD FOR YOUR WHOLE BODY
Bottled salad dressings
Palm oil
Standard olive oil

Bread Aisle
GOOD FOR YOUR WHOLE BODY
100% whole grain bread and pita
100% whole wheat English muffins
Tortillas, corn or whole wheat

NOT GOOD FOR YOUR WHOLE BODY

Bread labeled "wheat flour" that isn't 100% whole wheat
White bread
White flour tortilla

Cereal Aisle

GOOD FOR YOUR WHOLE BODY

Higher protein cereals, such as Kashi Go Rise, Special K
    Protein, or Kay's Naturals
Unsweetened oatmeal
Whole grain cereals (look for at least 3 grams of fiber and
    less than 5 grams of sugar per serving)

NOT GOOD FOR YOUR WHOLE BODY

Flavored, sweetened oatmeal
Granola bars

Snacks and Nuts

GOOD FOR YOUR WHOLE BODY

Dark chocolate (70% or higher cacao) chocolate
Multigrain crackers (look for 2 or more grams of fiber per
    serving)
Nuts (almonds, cashews, pistachios, walnuts)
Parmesan crisps
Popcorn

NOT GOOD FOR YOUR WHOLE BODY

Candy bars
Caramel corn
Crackers with more sugar than protein + fiber
Potato chips

Pasta, Grains, and Rice Aisle *(These can be found in boxes, microwave individual servings, and bulk section.)*

GOOD FOR YOUR WHOLE BODY

Barley

Brown rice

Buckwheat

Couscous

Farro

Pasta, whole wheat

Pulse pasta (such as chickpea and lentil)

Quinoa

NOT GOOD FOR YOUR WHOLE BODY

White rice

Canned and Packaged Goods

GOOD FOR YOUR WHOLE BODY

Beans, canned or dry (black, black-eyed, garbanzo, lentils, pinto)

Hummus

Packaged foods with more protein + fiber than sugar

NOT GOOD FOR YOUR WHOLE BODY

Baked beans with more sugar than protein + fiber

Packaged foods with more sugar than protein + fiber

Drinks

GOOD FOR YOUR WHOLE BODY

Coffee

Kombucha, unsweetened

Sparkling water

Teas (herbal and caffeinated)
Water flavored with "essence" (no calories)

NOT GOOD FOR YOUR WHOLE BODY

Sweetened energy or coffee drinks
Sweetened or diet soda
Sweetened teas

Condiments and Spices

GOOD FOR YOUR WHOLE BODY

Hot sauce and salsa
Kimchee
Sauerkraut, fermented, refrigerated
Spices
Vinegar: apple cider, balsamic, champagne, red wine

NOT GOOD FOR YOUR WHOLE BODY

An extra salt shaker

Frozen Foods *(Look for desserts that offer calcium and protein, then top them with healthy add-ons such as nuts and berries.)*

GOOD FOR YOUR WHOLE BODY

Frozen fruits
Frozen yogurt
Ice cream
Waffles, whole grain

NOT GOOD FOR YOUR WHOLE BODY

Cakes, cookies, pastries, and pudding
Waffles, white

Chapter 9

Take Your Whole Body Out to Eat

What to Eat (and Not Eat!) in All Your Favorite Restaurants (Yes, Even Fast Food!)

In an ideal world, every meal would be home-cooked, or thoughtfully prepared by chefs who had your health top of mind. In the real world, the tastebuds want what they want, and sometimes that means grabbing a quick meal out of a cardboard box or a clown's mouth, or at the place you and your best pals have met at for twenty years.

And this is where so many traditional eating plans fail us. If you're racing through town, hungry as a horse, and your local fast-food joint doesn't offer a meal that fits with your fancy zero-carb, coconut-oil-based, cauliflower-and-octopus-only fad diet, you're out of luck. That means you have to "break" your diet. That feels like failure, and it's one common reason that people often give up on fad diets.

That's not going to happen on this plan. You don't need to worry about specialty or forbidden foods; you just need to ensure you're getting the protein and fiber you need. While you can't always control for calories or sodium when you're dining out, you can hit the

143

Whole Body Reset nutritional guidelines almost anywhere you choose to dine. Just focus on getting at least 25 to 30 grams of protein and 5 grams of fiber. You'll be shocked to learn how many options are available, even at those fast-food outlets that have become synonymous with unhealthy eating.

We've scoured the menus of some of the most popular chain restaurants to find perfect Whole Body Reset combinations. Granted, many of them don't offer even unadulterated fruit to reach our four to six servings a day, so it never hurts to stick an apple or an orange in your bag or stash one in your car to have as a snack. If you don't see your go-to joint here, remember that at many restaurants you're usually safe ordering a green salad with protein, or a simple grilled piece of chicken or fish with vegetables and brown rice. A couple of popular fast-food joints didn't make the list, usually because there weren't any fiber-rich options on the menu. But again, if you're grabbing a burger at a chain not found here, add a fruit salad (if it's on the menu) or your own apple or orange for a quick dessert. In most cases, that will round out your meal and ensure that you're hitting both your protein and fiber needs. Remember: The Whole Body Reset is about more nutrition, not less food!

(Note: Menus are subject to change; often there are seasonal items that rotate and new items added, with some old ones dropped. Most chain restaurants offer the nutritional information of all their items online, and many include nutrition calculators that allow you to see the nutritional impact if you modify your selection.)

Applebee's

6 oz Select Sirloin + Fire-Grilled Veggies + Small Caesar Salad
41 g protein, 5 g fiber, 580 calories

Blackened Cajun Salmon + Garlicky Green Beans + Fire-Grilled Veggies + Fat-Free Italian Dressing
40 g protein, 8 g fiber, 580 calories

Arby's

Roast Buffalo Chicken + Curly Fries (snack size) + Side Salad
32 g protein, 7 g fiber, 680 calories

Roast Chicken Salad + Jalapeño Bites (5) + Side Salad
35 g protein, 6 g fiber, 610 calories

Au Bon Pain

Classic oatmeal (small) + Greek Vanilla Yogurt & Wild Blueberry Parfait (10.2 oz)
29 g protein, 8 g fiber, 490 calories

2 Eggs, Cheddar & Ham on Skinny Wheat Bagel
26 g protein, 7 g fiber, 350 calories

½ Tuna Salad Sandwich + Swiss Chard and Turkey Chili (large, 16 oz)
26 g protein, 21 g fiber, 450 calories

Mayan Chicken Harvest Hot Bowl
31 g protein, 7 g fiber, 670 calories

Boston Market

Turkey Breast (regular) + Bacon Brussels Sprouts + Cornbread
39 g protein, 7 g fiber, 560 calories

Buffalo Wild Wings

Brisket Tacos + Slaw
32 g protein, 6 g fiber, 630 calories

Six-count Traditional Wings with Signature Sauce + Carrots & Celery with Fat-Free Ranch
32 g protein, 3 g fiber, 313 calories

Burger King

Garden Chicken Salad with Crispy Chicken + ½ packet Ken's Lite Honey Balsamic Vinaigrette Dressing

25 g protein, 3 g fiber, 500 calories

(You'll need to add a piece of fruit to this meal for at least 2 more grams of fiber. See the list of options on page 347.)

Chick-fil-A

Egg White Grill + Sunflower Multigrain Bagel

33 g protein, 5 g fiber, 560 calories

Chik-fil-A Cool Wrap

42 g protein, 13 g fiber, 350 calories

Spicy Southwest Salad

33 g protein, 8 g fiber, 450 calories

Chili's

Chicken Enchilada Soup (bowl) + Lunch Combo House Salad + Ranch Dressing (1.5 oz)

24 g protein, 4 g fiber, 660 calories

6 oz Sirloin + Small Side of Fresh Guacamole + Side of Steamed Broccoli

38 g protein, 8 g fiber, 410 calories

Chipotle

Sofritas Burrito Bowl with light cilantro-lime brown rice, black beans, fajita vegetables, fresh tomato salsa, Monterey Jack cheese

27 g protein, 14 g fiber, 645 calories

Steak Salad with light cilantro-lime brown rice, light black beans, light Monterey Jack cheese, tomatillo red-chili salsa, chipotle honey vinaigrette dressing

31 g protein, 7.5 g fiber, 625 calories

Cracker Barrel Old Country Store

Cracker Barrel Country Boy Breakfast
27 g protein, 9 g fiber, 660 calories

Fresh Start Sampler + Turkey Sausage
35 g protein, 6 g fiber, 600 calories

Lemon-Grilled Rainbow Trout + Turnip Greens Bowl
67 g protein, 8 g fiber, 580 calories

Denny's

Loaded Veggie Omelet + Seasonal Fruit + English Muffin
34 g protein, 6 g fiber, 750 calories

Cobb Salad with Wild Alaskan Salmon and Light Italian Dressing
53 g protein, 6 g fiber, 790 calories

Dunkin'

Kosher Southwest Veggie Power Breakfast Sandwich
25 g protein, 5 g fiber, 420 calories

IHOP

2 Fried Eggs + Whole Wheat Toast + Turkey Sausage (2 pcs)
30 g protein, 5 g fiber, 410 calories

Chicken & Veggie Salad
38 g protein, 9 g fiber, 600 calories

55+ Turkey & Swiss Sandwich+ House Salad with ½ packet Balsamic Vinaigrette
45 g protein, 8 g fiber, 670 calories

Jack In the Box

Chicken Fajita Pita with Salsa + Side Salad + Low-Fat Balsamic Vinaigrette
28 g protein, 6 g fiber, 375 calories

Grilled Chicken Salad + Low-Fat Balsamic Vinaigrette

26 g protein, 7 g fiber, 500 calories

KFC

Crispy Colonel's Sandwich (Buffalo) + BBQ Baked Beans

35 g protein, 8 g fiber, 690 calories

Original Recipe Chicken Breast (on the bone) + Coleslaw

40 g protein, 6 g fiber, 560 calories

McDonald's

Premium Southwest Salad with Grilled Chicken

30 g protein, 6 g fiber, 320 calories

Olive Garden

Grilled Chicken Margherita (served with Parmesan Garlic Broccoli)

65 g protein, 6 g fiber, 540 calories

Herb-Grilled Salmon with Broccoli

49 g protein, 9 g fiber, 495 calories

Outback Steakhouse

Lobster Tail (5 oz) Steamed (served with fresh mixed veggies and seasoned rice) + Sweet Potato

32 g protein, 10 g fiber, 750 calories

Outback Center-Cut Sirloin (6 oz) + Fresh Steamed Broccoli

44 g protein, 5 g fiber, 360 calories

Steakhouse Salad

57 g protein, 7 g fiber, 750 calories

Panda Express

Vegetable Spring Roll (appetizer) + Honey Walnut Shrimp + Super Greens

22 g protein, 9 g fiber, 640 calories

String Bean Chicken Breast + half order fried rice + super greens
31 g protein, 10 g fiber, 540 calories

Panera Bread

Avocado, Egg White & Spinach on a Sprouted Grain Bagel Flat
(add bacon)
22 g protein, 5 g fiber, 420 calories

Green Goddess Cobb Salad with Chicken (whole)
41 g protein, 8 g fiber, 530 calories

Turkey on Rustic Sourdough (whole) + Ten Vegetable Soup (cup)
32 g protein, 4 g fiber, 470 calories

Popeyes

Bonafide Chicken Breast (1) + Corn on the Cob Cobbet (1)
35 g protein, 6 g fiber, 590 calories

Bonafide Chicken Leg (2 pcs) + Onion Rings (reg.) + Green Beans (reg.)
34 g protein, 7 g fiber, 653 calories

Catfish Filet (2 pcs) + Red Beans & Rice (reg.)
29 g protein, 7 g fiber, 707 calories

Starbucks

Hearty Blueberry Oatmeal + Spinach, Feta & Cage-Free Egg White
Breakfast Wrap
25 g protein, 8 g fiber, 510 calories

Chipotle Chicken Wrap Box
29 g protein, 8 g fiber, 630 calories

Subway

New Southwest Chicken Club*
34 g protein, 5 g fiber, 550 calories

Roast Beef Sub*

25 g protein, 6 g fiber, 290 calories

Turkey & Bacon Guacamole Sub*

49 g protein, 9 g fiber, 511 calories

 * All sandwich nutrients are based on 6-inch subs on 9-grain wheat bread with lettuce, tomatoes, green peppers, and cucumbers.

Steak Club Salad

45 g protein, 6 g fiber, 480 calories

Taco Bell

Power Menu Bowl (Chicken)

26 g protein, 7 g fiber, 470 calories

Steak Quesadilla + Black Beans & Rice

31 g protein, 8 g fiber, 690 calories

Texas Roadhouse

California Chicken Salad

78 g protein, 11 g fiber, 740 calories

Dallas Filet (6 oz) + Fire Roasted Green Chili Smother + Buttered Corn

50 g protein, 6 g fiber, 560 calories

Grilled Shrimp House Salad

65 g protein, 6 g fiber, 730 calories

Texas Red Chili (Bowl)

35 g protein, 6 g fiber, 490 calories

Wendy's

Apple Pecan Chicken Salad

39 g protein, 7 g fiber, 460 calories (add 60 calories per packet of dressing)

Chili (large) + half order Southwest Avocado Chicken Salad

43 g protein, 14 g fiber, 550 calories (add 80 calories per packet of dressing)

Parmesan Caesar Chicken Salad

49 g protein, 5 g fiber, 400 calories (add 80 calories per packet of dressing)

— ACTION STEP #9 —

Arm yourself before the next time you go out to eat: List what you eat at three favorite restaurants, and then write down a perfect Whole Body Reset meal you can create at each one. (Use our suggestions from this chapter, or find your own combos by checking the nutrition section of your go-to joint's website.) Don't forget that you can bring a piece of fruit or a small packet of nuts from home to add fiber and/or protein, and "cheat" your way to a perfect Whole Body Reset meal!

When I'm at _____ ,

I'll order _____

When I'm at _____ ,

I'll order _____

When I'm at _____ ,

I'll order _____

Chapter 10

Toss Out Your Old Diet Books

Why the Old Stand-By Plans Won't Work Anymore

In 1985, Wilford Brimley starred as an over-the-hill retiree who finds his vitality restored in the classic film *Cocoon*. He was fifty years old.

In 2022, Tom Cruise stars in, and does many of his own stunts for, his seventh *Mission: Impossible* film, as the hyperathletic secret agent Ethan Hunt. He will be sixty.

These two Hollywood anecdotes illustrate an important fact: We are simply a different generation than those who came before us, and we have wildly different expectations of what people our age should look like, feel like, and act like.

Remember the saying, "Life begins at forty"? That phrase dates back to the 1930s, popularized by a bestselling self-help book by psychologist Walter Pitkin. Today, forty feels more like a warm-up. We're still finding our footing when we hit that milestone. The late forties and beyond is where the action is; anybody who watched Jennifer Lopez (b. 1969) rock the 2020 Super Bowl halftime show, or appreciated Brad Pitt (b. 1963) baring his abs as a stuntman in *Once Upon a Time in . . . Hollywood*, or enjoyed Meryl Streep (b. 1949) sliding down the banister in *Mamma Mia! Here We Go Again* knows that we don't need an invasion of *Cocoon*-like alien eggs to restore our youthful powers. All we need is the knowledge of how to feed and care for our bodies, and the motivation to see it through.

And yet . . . smart nutritional guidelines and effective weight-management programs for people our age are still difficult to come by. Why?

Dumbest Diet Ideas Ever (Yes, These Are Real)

Struggles with weight can cause us to make questionable choices. And there's no shortage of hucksters out there who would be happy to supply gimmicky solutions, knowing that no matter how wacky they may sound, someone, somewhere, might just pay for them. Here are a few that people actually fell for, in descending order of difficulty and/or disgustingness.

Baby Food Diet. Supposedly created by a celebrity trainer, this diet proposes that you replace two meals a day with, yes, jars of baby food. Beyond the obvious lack of flavor, or common sense, involved in this diet, the impact on your social life—assuming you're not in day care—is gonna be pretty severe.

Fletcherizing Diet. Devised by guy named Horace Fletcher after he was denied health insurance because of his obesity, this plan lets you eat whatever you want, whenever you want. The catch: Whatever you put into your mouth, you have to chew until it turns completely to liquid, then "drink" it down. Just imagine how much chewing it would take to turn Mom's pot roast into pot roast juice.

Where the Confusion Starts

A lot happened in the year 1980: John Lennon, patron saint of '60s idealism, was murdered, and Ronald Reagan, patron saint of the modern conservative movement, was elected president. CNN launched, ushering in the era of 24-hour news, and we were all riveted by TV coverage of the Iranian hostage crisis, the eruption of Mount St. Helens, and the U.S. Olympic hockey team's nearly impossible "Miracle on Ice."

Clay Diet. Popularized by an actress who had to portray an anorexic/bulimic, this one involves stirring clay into a glass of water and drinking it down. The diet supposedly cleanses you of toxins, but it also deprives you of necessary nutrients.

Air Diet. Mmm, can you taste the apple pie? The chocolate brownie sundae? The Philly cheesesteak? Yes, you can, if you use your imagination, since following this diet involves only pretending to eat food, when what you're actually eating is nothing but air.

Tapeworm Diet. In some corners of the dark web, you can order capsules filled with tapeworm eggs. Swallow them, and in addition to ingesting a parasite, you've also put yourself at risk for endless bouts of debilitating pain, nausea, and diarrhea, as well as possible organ failure and dementia. We all love having a dinner companion, but ideally, that companion would not actually be inside your body.

Bottom line: If it involves eating something weird, or eating in a weird way, it's not a healthy or sustainable approach to managing your weight. Let common sense be your guide.

And while all that was going on, another watershed moment slipped quietly into American society that year: Two government agencies, the U.S. Department of Agriculture (USDA) and the Department of Health and Human Services (HHS), jointly released a twenty-page pamphlet called *Nutrition and Your Health: Dietary Guidelines for Americans.*

The guidelines were pretty simple, listing five major food groups (fruits and vegetables; grains; meats, poultry, fish, and eggs; legumes; and dairy), and it would be hard to argue with any of its original seven dietary directives: "Eat a variety of foods," "Avoid too much sugar," that sort of thing.

Every five years since then, the USDA and HHS have issued a revised set of guidelines, each growing longer and more complex. The original food groups became a food pyramid, then a food plate. While you've probably never read the *Dietary Guidelines for Americans,* you can be sure it affects your life. Educators, nutritionists, and policymakers use its guidelines to make recommendations and guide federally funded food programs (remember the "ketchup is a vegetable" school lunch controversy?), while manufacturers update their package labels (and health claims) to reflect the latest recommendations. With each update, institutions from schools to senior centers adjust their menus, and those Nutrition Facts panels you find on packages in the grocery store get a refresh. (And, as we saw in Chapter 8, those informative panels can be effective tools in helping us suss out which packaged foods belong in our grocery carts.)

But as explained in the Introduction to this book, the *Dietary Guidelines* now *includes* specific Recommended Daily Allowances (RDAs) for each age category: for toddlers, teens, young adults, and folks in their twenties and thirties and forties, broken out by gender, and carefully curated up to age fifty. But there, the *Dietary Guidelines*—which outlined our changing nutritional requirements through the first half-century of life—suddenly becomes nonspecific. Which means that we're no longer getting the detailed, decade-by-decade information we need to make smart choices.

How the *Dietary Guidelines* Shortchanges Us

Given what we know about our changing bodies and our changing nutritional needs, we can see three distinct areas where people at midlife need to diverge from these guidelines. And here's where the Whole Body Reset becomes so important.

Protein

The *Dietary Guidelines* assigns the same RDAs for everyone over the age of eighteen—about 46 grams of protein per day for women and 56 grams per day for men. But our changing bodies lose muscle faster and digest protein less efficiently, as we discussed in Chapter 1. So while those numbers may be sensible recommendations for people looking to maintain general health in their twenties, thirties, and early forties, they're dramatically lower than what our bodies need as we age. "I'm very comfortable saying that the RDA for protein is probably too low for older people," Katherine Tucker told me. Tucker sits on the Food and Nutrition Board of the National Academies of Sciences, Engineering, and Medicine, which develops the RDAs. She says it will be several years before government guidelines can catch up to current research. The *Dietary Guidelines* also indicates nothing about protein timing and the science that shows having adequate amounts at each meal is crucial for older adults.

So the problems that plague the 2020–2025 *Dietary Guidelines* may exist well into the future. The protein recommendation remains low, while people our age will continue to struggle with issues related to weight gain and muscle loss.

Fiber

The *Dietary Guidelines* recommends that women 50+ drop their fiber intake from 25 to 22 grams a day, men from 31 grams per day down to 28 grams. But to lose weight, eating *30* grams of fiber per day was nearly as effective as cutting out sugar, fat, salt, AND alcohol, according to a recent study of people with metabolic syndrome (those with a combination of health factors including high cholesterol, blood pressure, and blood sugar, and excess belly fat). And in another study, an extra 10 grams of fiber per 1,000 calories predicted a reduction of about 4.3 years in biologic aging. The researcher, from Brigham Young University, looked at more than 5,600 U.S. adults and found a link between fiber intake and longer telomeres, which are strands of nucleotides that help protect your DNA from damage and may help to forecast how long you'll live.[1]

The recommendation of less fiber is in part a function of the reduced calories that the *Dietary Guidelines* advises. It suggests that women and men cut about 200 calories per day out of their diets after age fifty. But reducing calories shouldn't mean reducing nutrition! Instead, we should switch to a diet higher in fruit and vegetables to compensate for a slowing metabolism (which, as we point out in Chapter 2, may be based more on myth than science) that would naturally lead to an increased intake of fiber. Many people experience bloating or other side effects when they eat too much fiber, but in most cases 30 grams per day should not be an issue.

Vitamins

As we age, our ability to absorb and utilize B vitamins changes as well, primarily due to the changes in our digestive systems—we manufacture less stomach acid, reducing our ability to pull these vitamins out of our food. Vitamin B12 becomes harder for us to access, while B6 deficiencies are common as well. So, logically, we'd have to eat more of these nutrients to get the same benefit that we did when we were in our thirties. But the guidelines don't yet recommend increased B12, despite the fact that one national survey found that more than 16 percent of older adults have low vitamin B12 concentrations in their blood. Vitamin B6 intake does get a little bit of a boost from the USDA, from 1.3 milligrams per day for both men and women to 1.5 milligrams daily for females over age fifty, and 1.7 milligrams for men over that age.

Fortunately, some smart guidelines for people over fifty do exist. MyPlate for Older Adults, created by Tufts University in conjunction with AARP Foundation, takes much of the guessing out of the USDA's guidelines and shows how to eat proportionately at every meal. It's a good visual guideline to what a standard meal should look like, and whereas the *Dietary Guidelines* just gives nutrition totals, MyPlate for Older Adults breaks down those nutrients into actual foods you might eat at meals. As long as you remember to build on the MyPlate recommendations by making sure you get 25 to 30 grams of protein at each meal (particularly breakfast), you can't go wrong.

Why Most Diet Plans Don't Lead to Permanent Weight Loss

While government guidelines for protein and fiber may be less than optimal, the diet industry offers no end of additional, sometimes confounding, often contradictory, and sometimes downright crazy nutritional advice. And most popular eating plans—even if they're relatively solid in terms of their overall contribution to wellness—fail to address the way our bodies change as we age.

From Atkins to Paleo to South Beach, most diets are created for the general public. But they don't take into consideration the needs of the mature physique. Here, we'll look at some of the most influential diets of the last few decades and explain why our bodies need something different.

Keto Diet and Intermittent Fasting

Maybe you know someone who snarfs down piles of bacon but thinks toast is evil. Perhaps you have friends who won't go to dinner after 7 p.m. because the time falls outside their "food window."

These behaviors are all linked to popular weight-loss programs that share a common approach: to make your body achieve ketosis, a metabolic state that switches your body's engine from sugar burner to fat burner. But ketosis happens naturally for most of us, every day; after about six hours of not eating (during which we're probably asleep), the body naturally begins using fat for energy, says Pamela Peeke, MD, Pew Foundation Scholar in Nutrition and Metabolism and assistant professor of Medicine at the University of Maryland.

The "keto diet" tries to trick the body into ketosis for longer periods by limiting the amount of protein one eats (to about 15 percent of calories) and consuming no more than 50 grams of carbs a day—about as much as you'd get in a serving of rice and beans, a couple of apples, or two ears of corn.

Keto is a great example of a diet that may seem to work for some

---

What Is "Bulletproof Coffee"?

Ever see someone drinking regular joe with a pat of butter and some oil mixed in? The concept behind what's known as Bulletproof Coffee and its wide-ranging franchise is much the same as keto: nothing but coffee and some fat in the morning to trigger ketosis in the first half of the day. But by depriving your body of the protein it needs, this diet idea may help accelerate age-related muscle loss.

people but is absolutely inappropriate for people at midlife and older. The biggest risk of keto dieting is that you're often depriving your body of the protein it needs to build and maintain muscle mass. By limiting yourself to 20 percent of calories from protein, you're automatically falling short of what you need to maintain muscle mass— and setting yourself up for eventual rebound weight gain, as well as a long-term risk of falls and fractures. In addition, carbs—in the forms of fruits, vegetables, legumes, and whole grains—are where we get a vast array of nutrients, including fiber, vitamins, minerals, and phytonutrients. And reducing nutrition at this stage of the game just isn't good dietary advice.

And while some studies have shown ketogenic diets to be effective for weight loss, that's in part because, as Carla Prado, an associate professor of nutrition at the University of Alberta in Edmonton, says: "The diet is very monotonous. There just isn't much that you can eat, so you wind up eating less." When government researchers designed a study to hold calorie intakes constant, they found no advantage to keto versus a balanced diet with carbohydrates. Plus, much of what people lose in keto is, at least initially, water weight. Here's why: Sugar stored in your body (glycogen) is bound with H_2O. So when you start cutting carbs, your body grabs that sugar for energy and releases the water. What appears to be fat loss is, in fact, a rapid loss of water.

There's another trend that's linked to the idea of ketosis: intermittent fasting. It comes in many different styles and permutations: One approach calls for dramatically cutting calories on regular days throughout the week (known as the 5:2 Diet—five days on, two off). The idea here is to eat no more than 500 calories on fasting days, and to eat normally during the rest of the week. Then there's time-restricted eating, in which you're only allowed to eat for a period of four or six or eight hours out of every twenty-four. In most cases, the idea is to skip, or at least delay, breakfast and/or lunch, then close the kitchen by 8 p.m. or earlier. And finally, for the hardcore who really want to play Hunger Games, there's complete fasting for twenty-four-hour periods.

A study in mice found that intermittent fasting had some particular health and aging benefits, but those findings haven't been duplicated in humans at midlife and beyond. When it comes to weight management, however, intermittent fasting is just another way of restricting calories; there's nothing magical about it, regardless of what method one chooses. (I've watched intermittent fasters scarf down a day's worth of food at one sitting.) Intermittent fasting works no better or worse than a traditional calorie-restrictive diet,[2] according to a review of eleven different trials.

Worse, a small study in *The Journal of the American Medical Association (JAMA)* found that intermittent fasting was harder for people to stick to than traditional diets.[3] Which makes sense: Hunger signals can be distracting, not to mention miserable. And meals don't just "fuel" our bodies; they're social events, whether it's checking in with your partner at the breakfast table, networking with colleagues over lunch, or meeting friends for dinner at the end of the day. And who wants to drop their relationships just to drop a few pounds?

And while you're losing relationships, you may also be losing muscle: Another *JAMA* study published in 2020 found that time-restricted eating "could exacerbate muscle loss."[4]

That said, there is a solid argument for setting a reasonable cutoff time for eating, at least on most days, according to Peeke. "What's happening today with people fifty and older is their diets are a chaotic mess," Peeke told me. "We eat when we feel like eating, we get into rotten habits like Netflixing late into the night with snacks." In a study[5] she conducted, when people cut their eating time to just twelve hours a day—starting breakfast at 8 a.m., say, and finishing their last meal by 8 p.m.—they naturally lose about eleven pounds over the course of four weeks. The reason is that giving your body that twelve-hour break between meals extends the ketosis process naturally—without draconian restrictions or having to turn healthy carbs and muscle-protecting proteins into an enemy. Peeke recommends making twelve hours of not eating your go-to approach, but maybe tweaking that to ten hours of eating and fourteen hours of not eating on days when your schedule allows.

BOTTOM LINE: We need protein throughout the day, which these programs often forbid. You can "fast" simply by limiting your eating to twelve hours a day or less, but otherwise, leave keto and fasting to the crash dieters.

The Mediterranean Diet

The Mediterranean diet is consistently ranked as the healthiest diet in the world by the *U.S. News and World Report*. And for good reason: It lowers the risk of heart disease and overall death in people who had coronary heart disease, according to a 2018 study. Equally important, it may slow the decline of mental acuity as well as the growth of beta-amyloid deposits, a marker of Alzheimer's disease.

There's no one exact Mediterranean diet—if there were, French, Italian, Lebanese, and Greek restaurants would all offer the same food. Instead, it more reflects an approach to eating based on whole grains, fruits and vegetables, olive oil, and seafood; moderate amounts of yogurt, eggs, milk, and lean meats like poultry; reduced red meat consumption; and far fewer sweets and processed foods than Americans typically eat.

Sounds a lot like the Whole Body Reset? Yep! Both approaches advocate reducing junk food; focusing on healthy oils and high-fiber fruits, vegetables, and grains; and making lean meats, dairy, and seafood our primary sources of protein. The primary difference, in fact, is simply timing: Ideally, you'd be eating in a Mediterranean style while still being sure to eat quality protein and fiber in the morning and afternoon as well as at night, to keep your muscle maintenance in high gear.

BOTTOM LINE: Follow the Mediterranean way of eating and you may reduce your risk of heart disease and other conditions. But make sure you spread adequate fiber and protein throughout the day.

The DASH Diet

No, this is not a diet in which you eat an expensive meal at a restaurant and then run out the door before the check comes. "DASH" in this instance stands for Dietary Approaches to Stop Hypertension, and it was developed by the National Institutes of Health to help people lower their blood pressure without the use of medications. Its primary approach is to help you lower your sodium intake while increasing the amount of heart-healthy potassium, calcium, and magnesium you take in. These minerals are critical to relaxing the blood vessels and counteracting the effects of sodium.

DASH—another top-ranked diet—is very similar to the Mediterranean diet. DASH emphasizes fruits, vegetables, nuts, seeds, legumes, and whole grains; allows moderate amounts of dairy and lean meats, although you'll eat less seafood than on the Mediterranean diet; and limits sweets to just five or fewer servings per week. And like the Mediterranean diet, DASH can help reduce the risk of heart disease and may reduce the risk of age-related dementia, according to the Alzheimer's Association.

When the Mayo Clinic put together a sample daily menu on the DASH diet, it came out looking a lot like the Whole Body Reset, with 90 grams of protein, 39 grams of fiber, and plenty of heart-healthy monounsaturated fats. But the DASH diet doesn't emphasize proteins throughout the day, and that's a real failing for us grown-ups who want not only healthy hearts, but healthy muscles and bones as well.

BOTTOM LINE: As the DASH diet recommends, the best dietary approach to reducing high blood pressure is to cut down on sodium

Beware of Hidden Treasures

More fruits, vegetables, dairy, legumes, and nuts are going to lead automatically to more calcium, potassium, and magnesium. That's great. But cutting salt—that once-valued treasure—is harder. According to the Centers for Disease Control and Prevention, the number one source of sodium in the American diet isn't the salt shaker; nor is it potato chips and French fries.

It's bread.

In fact, "breads and rolls" is number one and "sandwiches" is number three on the list of sodium sources. Pizza, cold cuts and cured meats, and soups round out the top five. White sandwich bread in particular tends to be high in salt: A single slice of bread, for example, can give you 230 milligrams of sodium, which is 10 percent of all the sodium you're allowed per day by the *Dietary Guidelines*. A 2018 study named dozens of bread brands, from Whole Foods to Nature's Own, as particularly high in sodium. Yes, you can still enjoy a sandwich, but you might want to reconsider that enticing basket of fresh rolls while waiting for your meal to arrive, and vary your starches with sweet potatoes, brown rice, and whole wheat pastas.

and processed foods and to eat more fruits, vegetables, and dairy. But if you're watching your salt intake, read labels when you shop, and beware of sneaky sources of sodium.

The MIND Diet

Think of the MIND diet as a mash up of the Mediterranean and DASH diets, with a specific focus on foods that are particularly effective in promoting brain health. Research indicates that the MIND diet is effective in slowing age-related cognitive decline, and in the best case scenario, helping your brain perform as though it were 7.5 years younger.

Like the Whole Body Reset, the MIND diet emphasizes leafy green vegetables, berries, nuts, olive oil, seafood, and beans.

BOTTOM LINE: Much like the Mediterranean and DASH approaches, MIND is a healthy way of eating that easily conforms to the Whole Body Reset approach. But again, be mindful (pun intended!) of getting enough high-fiber foods and spreading your protein throughout the day.

The Blue Zones

Move more. Stress less. Love your friends and family. Eat more plants.

There are few recommendations from the Blue Zones Project that anyone can object to. The Blue Zones Project came from a study of areas of the world where people tend to live longer—places in the Mediterranean, such as Ikaria, Greece, and the Ogliastra region of Sardinia; Okinawa, Japan; Loma Linda, California; and the Nicoya Peninsula in Costa Rica. In each place, people tended to eat plant-based, Mediterranean-style diets; enjoy moderate exercise; and maintain close social ties.

The results of this lifestyle can be striking: In Loma Linda, where the highest population of Seventh-day Adventists lives, some people enjoy an average of ten additional healthy years of life compared to the average American.

BOTTOM LINE: Eating more plants—which means more vitamins and minerals and fiber—is a great way to improve almost any diet. But note that "plant-based" is not necessarily "plants only." Following the Whole Body Reset will naturally up your intake of these Blue Zone foods while also ensuring you're getting enough protein throughout the day to stay lean and strong. And because the Whole Body Reset requires no weird time restrictions, forbidden foods, or expensive specialty items, you'll be likely to follow one particularly welcome recommendation of the Blue Zones approach: to share the Whole Body Reset experience with friends and family.

Paleo

The general concept behind the Paleo diet is that we evolved as hunter-gatherers, and so we should eat in that manner—focusing on game meats, fish, and plants that can grow wild, while eschewing not only processed foods but grains such as wheat, rice, and corn; beans, lentils, and peanuts; dairy foods such as milk, yogurt, and cheese; and other products of modern agriculture.

In fact, though, most of what we're sold as "Paleo" bears little if any resemblance to what our ancient ancestors ate. Wild plants and animals are simply different from what's available in the grocery store today. In fact, if you really want to follow a Paleo diet, go out into your backyard, turn over a rock, and eat whatever comes crawling out. Because as mighty as those ancient hunters may have been in bringing down woolly mammoths, in reality insects—especially grubs, caterpillars, and grasshoppers—probably made up a considerable part of their protein intake. Oh, and you'll need to up your fiber intake a bit more as well: Ancient humans may have eaten up to 100 grams of fiber per day, according to some research, because wild plants tend to be more fibrous than today's cultivated versions.

But let's say you were able to stay clear of the grocery store and live only on what you could hunt or forage. Does following an ancient diet help you live longer and more healthfully? It's hard to tell, since few Paleo people made it into their later years. But interestingly, a 2013 study of 137 mummies from hunter-gatherer societies around the world (average age at death: forty-three) found that a third of them showed signs of atherosclerosis.

BOTTOM LINE: Cutting out processed foods and sweets? That makes sense. Cutting out healthy foods such as whole grains, dairy, and beans? No. Too many studies have shown the importance of these foods in maintaining overall health and keeping our weight under control. And as for the bugs . . . well, that's up to you.

The Whole30

For thirty days, you give up sugar (sounds good), alcohol (can't hurt), grains and legumes (uh-oh), and dairy (oh boy).

As with other "phase" diets, the Whole30 is designed to crash your system with a massive reduction in carbohydrates, while also eliminating foods you might be sensitive to (like alcohol, gluten from wheat, or lactose from dairy). You eat only lean meats, eggs, and seafood; fruits and vegetables; and healthy sources of fat such as nuts and avocados. By the end of the thirty days, you'll have hopefully dropped pounds and identified some unhealthy foods that you can start living without.

As with any elimination diet, especially one that cuts out carbs, the Whole30 will probably cause you to drop a few pounds in water weight quickly. And any diet that restricts what you can eat or when you can eat will give you, at least temporarily, a sense of control over your food intake. But there's no scientific evidence that this approach will result in long-term weight loss.

Plus, eliminating both dairy and high-fiber grains and legumes means you're dramatically cutting your intake of calcium, fiber, and gut-healthy probiotics, all necessary for lowering inflammation, improving heart health, and regulating immune function. It also makes it nearly impossible to follow a plant-based diet, because it cuts out the most nutritious plant foods around—traditional healthy foods such as tofu and rice and beans.

BOTTOM LINE: The Whole30 is a classic crash diet that you "go on" and then "go off." It's not a sustainable way of eating. If you're interested in eliminating certain food groups to see if they're causing bloating or other physical issues, it makes sense to consult your doctor first. Experts sometimes recommend eliminating foods one by one, rather than all together.

Atkins/South Beach/Low-Carb Diets

Atkins and the South Beach diet are among the most popular of the low-carb diets. And since many of the carbs we eat today are refined (white rice, white bread, pretzels, crackers), fried in oil (potato chips, corn chips, fries), and loaded with sugar (cookies, candy, cakes, muffins), cutting down dramatically on carbs makes an awful lot of sense. But those diets begin to make a lot less sense when you're cutting down on fruits, vegetables, and whole grains, an unfortunate aspect of both programs.

Atkins and South Beach both rely on a gimmick called "phases." In Atkins, for example, you start by cutting carbs down to just 20 grams a day, most of it from vegetables such as celery, cucumber, and asparagus, while eating protein and fat at every meal—but you eliminate most fruits, nuts, and grains. This phase lasts for at least two weeks, after which you're allowed some fruits and seeds until you come within ten pounds of your eventual weight-loss goal, at which point the diet begins to become a bit more forgiving. The South Beach diet follows a similar format: No fruits or grains for the first two weeks, although you can add back some fruits and whole grains after that initial period.

Diet plans that use phases are designed to trigger quick, noticeable weight loss. But as we now know, the first thing that happens when you cut carbs is that your body releases stored water; much of the initial weight loss is really just water loss. And studies show that when people lose weight rapidly, they typically gain back about half of it within two years, and about 80 percent of the weight within five years.[6] The Whole Body Reset, on the other hand, is a way of life, a long-term lifestyle solution, designed to change not just your food but your vitality—physical, mental, and emotional.

But more important, when we cut out whole grains, we lose some important B vitamins—vitamins our bodies are already having trouble accessing because of our changing digestive system. When we cut out fruits, we reduce our intake of thousands of phytochemicals that our bodies need to help fight advancing inflammation. And cutting both whole grains and fruit causes our intake of fiber to drop. While the high-protein emphasis of plans like this are useful for those of us in middle age who are concerned about holding on to muscle mass, protein is only one part of our battle plan against age-related muscle loss. We also need to pack our days with high-fiber, high-nutrition

If Food's Got You Beat

A friend in her late fifties has been a yo-yo dieter since grade school. No matter the diet, she couldn't stick to it. Food called out to her relentlessly, and she lost the battle daily. Finally she heard about Overeaters Anonymous (similar to Alcoholics Anonymous) and tried it. "OA doesn't give you a specific food plan," she explains. "It just helps you stop crazy food behaviors. For the first time in my life, I can eat sanely." Learn more at oa.org.

Chronic overeating, eating compulsion, binging, purging, and restricting can all be symptoms of an eating disorder. Reach out to the National Eating Disorder Association to find help near where you live (nationaleatingdisorders.org).

Another option is to work with a qualified professional who can help you tailor a food plan that works for you. You can search for experts who offer in-person and virtual guidance at eatright.org.

foods that help to support our immune systems, reduce inflammation, and turn back the tide of premature aging. And that's where many of these programs can fall short.

BOTTOM LINE: "Low carb" often means "low nutrition." Aim for a protein-rich diet that also arms you with the vitamins and minerals your body craves, and avoid diets that offer gimmicky phases and quick, temporary results.

Noom and Cognitive Behavioral Therapy

Noom is a cuddly, app-based weight-loss program that's grounded in the principles of cognitive behavioral therapy—where you learn to listen and talk back to your negative thoughts. Join Noom, for a fee (sometimes a free trial, so long as you hand over your credit card), and you begin by building a lifestyle and psychological profile designed to help you overcome the emotional barriers that prevent weight loss and lead to overeating. This approach is designed to help keep you on track and feeling supported in your weight-loss journey. Can't argue with that.

The food aspect of the program, however, comes down to a very simple strategy: Eat less calorie-dense food. And the way you do that is to reduce fat (by eating low-fat dairy instead of full-fat dairy, or by choosing air-popped popcorn over fried chips), or to eat foods with more water in them (grapes instead of raisins, salads instead of burgers).

That's not a bad strategy at all, especially if you're aggressively choosing fruits and vegetables over burgers and fries. And by emphasizing sustainability over rapid weight loss, Noom takes a healthy, long-term approach that's designed to minimize the yo-yo dieting effect. But there are three problems with the Noom approach that make it less than ideal for people at midlife and beyond.

First, there's the focus on weight. Noom wants you to weigh

yourself every day, putting the emphasis on body size, not shape. As a result, there's no real way to tell if that weight loss is from a reduction in water weight, a loss of muscle tissue, or actual fat loss. And as we know, the scale tells only one part of the story.

Second, there's no real acknowledgment of how our bodies change as we age. While the profiling aspect really helps you work through your food issues, keeps you focused on your goals, and challenges your existing misconceptions, the prescriptive aspect of the program is pretty standard: Eat fewer calories. And because protein sources tend to contain fat, and hence be more calorie-dense, there's a real danger that protein may get the short shrift. In the end, weight loss + less protein = muscle loss, and we've already learned just how unhealthy that can be.

Finally, while cognitive behavioral therapy has proven effective in treating binge-eating disorders, its efficacy in terms of weight loss for the average person is not as clear.

BOTTOM LINE: Knowing what to eat is one thing; actually eating what you know to be healthy is something different. The Whole Body Reset is designed as a very simple, lifelong approach to eating that can and will deliver results by reducing hunger and packing in nutrition. But for those who find themselves mindlessly snacking in ways they can't control, cognitive behavioral therapies may be a useful addition to a well-balanced diet program.

Throughout this chapter, you've no doubt spotted a couple of familiar themes: First, dietary guidelines and most modern diet programs don't take into consideration the specific needs of people in midlife and beyond. Second, a lot of weight-loss programs are geared toward short-term results at the expense of long-term wellness. No wonder we've spent most of our lives confused about what to eat, when to eat, and how to eat.

But there is something we can do—something that is good for the long haul. It's not a fad. It's a nutrition and weight-management program designed for OUR bodies, one that is easy to do today and every day, one that addresses and even reverses some of the effects of aging while stopping weight gain in its tracks and setting us back on the path to a leaner, healthier, longer life.

It is, of course, the Whole Body Reset.

— ACTION STEP #10 —

When stress or boredom hits, it's hard to make smart food choices. That's why they call it "comfort food."

If eating when you're stressed or bored is one of your major obstacles, try writing down your go-to unhealthy escapes, and then, at right, list a healthier alternative or upgrade. For example, if you tend to snack on potato chips, what about corn chips and guacamole? Or if you tend to grab a handful of pretzels, try getting the same crunch from carrot sticks and hummus. This program isn't about eating less food. It's about eating more nutrition.

My Stress Go-To   **My Healthy Swap**

_____   _____

_____   _____

_____   _____

Slowing down and eating more mindfully, and trying other coping activities such as deep breathing, listening to music, and meditating can be helpful alternatives when we're eating because of stress or boredom instead of hunger.

Chapter 11

The Metabolism Myth

Exercise Isn't Great for Weight Loss
(It's True!) So Why Should We Do It?

Wait, what? What did we just say? Exercise isn't great for weight loss?

That's right—at least, not in the way we think it is. Exercise doesn't "burn" calories—at least not in the way we think it does. It doesn't dramatically cause you to lose weight, and it doesn't "boost" your metabolism. Indeed, pretty much everything you've been told about the value of exercise is wrong.

Let's say you're that average person in his or her fifties, and yesterday, you woke up late, went to work, ate lunch at your desk, then came home and watched TV all night. In that case, your body burned about 2,500 calories.

Today, you got up early, spent half an hour on the treadmill, worked all day, and took an hour-long yoga class before dinner. Today, your body burned about 2,500 calories.

All that extra activity, and not a whit of calorie-burning impact.

How is this possible? What about those cool digital readouts on the stair-climbing machine that tell us we burned hundreds of calories in each sweat session? Well, it's true that our bodies expend a lot of calories during exercise. The problem is, our daily metabolism is pretty set; if we burn more calories exercising, our bodies compensate.

"When you exercise more, your body simply lowers the number of calories it burns performing other functions, such as inflammation or hormone production," researcher Herman Pontzer told me. The associate professor of evolutionary anthropology at Duke University and author of *Burn: New Research Blows the Lid Off How We Really Burn Calories, Lose Weight, and Stay Healthy* explains, "So the

---

Burn Calories, Stay Healthy, and Lose Weight

Our bodies do best with a minimum of 150 minutes a week of moderate-intensity aerobic physical activity (or 75 minutes a week of vigorous-intensity exercise), according to the Centers for Disease Control and Prevention. That's about 30 minutes of moderate exercise five days a week or 20 minutes of vigorous exercise four days a week. And that activity can be spread throughout the day.

Does 30 minutes sound like a lot? It's not. In fact, 30 minutes is . . .

- about one-tenth the amount of time the average Baby Boomer spends on a smartphone every single day.
- one-sixth of the amount of time the average American spends watching TV each day.

The fact is, you can do much of what's suggested here while catching up on the latest Netflix sensation, rocking to your favorite beat, or listening to an audio book or podcast. Or grab a workout buddy or find a group—in person or remote—and get stronger together.

---

number of calories you burn per day—your metabolism—remains constant, whether you work out or no."

It's true.

Pontzer came about these findings in part by studying primitive cultures, such as the Hadza tribe in Tanzania. The Hadza hunt their food with simple tools and build their huts from grass; because they work day and night for survival, scientists assumed they must burn a lot of calories. But when Pontzer measured their metabolic rates, he discovered that the average Hadza burns no more calories in a day than the average American couch potato.

Perhaps you've read about workouts or even diets that are designed to "boost" your metabolism. Malarky, Pontzer says. Think about it from an evolutionary standpoint: Our metabolism is set by the number of calories we need to survive. If we turned up our metabolism, we'd be increasing our risk of starvation. So nature protects us from that by keeping our metabolic rate constant, in spite of our attempts to burn calories through exercise.

Unfortunately, that starts to change as we age and begin to lose muscle mass and gain fat; as we mentioned earlier in this book, muscle is simply more metabolically active than fat.

There's more news, and it's not good news: If we do indeed face a dramatic shortage of calories, our bodies are capable of turning our metabolic rates down, causing us to burn fewer calories. That way, we're protected from times of famine. Which is great, unless the "famine" is artificially manufactured by a calorie-reduction diet. Deprive yourself of enough calories, and you reset your metabolic rate lower—which sets you up for future weight gain.

In fact, that's exactly what happens when we follow a traditional diet, one that restricts calories and, in many cases, leads to muscle loss. (It's one of the reasons a study of fourteen *Biggest Loser* contestants, conducted by the National Institutes of Health, found that thirteen of them had gained a significant amount of the weight back within six years. On average, the resting metabolic rate for contestants was 1,900 calories a day—down from an average of 2,607 before they started their diet.)

That's why the Whole Body Reset doesn't ask you to restrict calories dramatically. In the long run, restricting calories causes weight gain! Instead, we only lightly tweak your normal eating patterns, shifting to a higher protein content (for muscle maintenance and hunger reduction), more fiber and high-nutrient foods (to battle inflammation), and less junk. When you follow the Whole Body Reset, you may eat slightly fewer calories than you burn each day, but only slightly—and you'll still eat enough to keep your metabolism at its normal, healthy pace.

Why Exercise Matters

So, if exercise doesn't cause us to burn additional calories, why should we do it?

Because you are an athlete. And an athlete is always training.

Yes, this means you.

Every day, when you get out of bed, you set about training your body. Just as Tom Brady makes choices that train him to play the position of quarterback—practicing to throw a football and dodge lunging tacklers—so, too, do you make daily choices that train your body to do certain things.

And both you and Brady face serious dangers from your chosen lifestyles. Brady can get crushed by a linebacker or damage a knee trying to sprint to safety. The dangers that you face, on the other hand, come along less suddenly. Sitting for long periods—be it at a desk, behind the wheel, or in a comfy chair—can cause muscles such as the hamstrings (the long muscles at the back of your thighs) to atrophy, while increasing your risk of peripheral vascular disease and blood clots. Meanwhile, the discs in your back are slowly compressed, leading to an increased risk of back pain.

Over time, too much sitting can lead to higher cholesterol, higher blood pressure, and higher blood sugar.[1] In fact, studies show that sitting all day with no physical activity is as hazardous to your health as obesity and smoking. And we already know how age can take a toll on our muscular strength, and just how dangerous that can be for our overall well-being.

Which is why, as an athlete, you need to train your body.

"What we call 'exercise' isn't different from your daily life," explains Jay Cardiello, personal trainer in New York City and co-founder of Off the Scale, Mt. Sinai Hospital's obesity and disease intervention program. "Exercise is simply adapting your daily life into different positions and different stressors. If you're behind a desk all day, that's your field of play; you have to train to meet that daily challenge."

But training your body in a different way—by adding moderately intense exercise—can reduce the risks of too much sitting, just as training to improve his quickness and agility helps Brady reduce the risks of getting smeared across the football field. These ideas—not "weight loss"—explain why exercise is important, and these are the ideas that inform Your Whole Body Fitness Plan, the program that begins in the next chapter.

You're already using elements of fitness in your daily life—elements like strength, power, speed, endurance, flexibility—and the more you simply move during the day, the healthier you'll be. You test your fitness when you run to catch a closing elevator, lift and carry your grocery bags, pull open the refrigerator door, bend to pick up something you dropped, or just scratch your own back. Training will help you do all you want to do with more ease and grace.

By "training," we mean three different things:

The first is strength training, also called resistance training, which helps you build and retain muscle.

The second is cardio training, which will keep your heart and lungs strong. Strength and cardio training are like peanut butter and jelly. They're both good. But doing them both is unbeatable.

A variation on these two is high intensity interval training, or HIIT, which is a clever, if demanding, way of combing strength and cardio for maximum benefit.

Beyond muscular and cardiovascular fitness, you're going to be focusing on a third aspect of overall physical health: balance and flexibility, an area that even avid exercisers often ignore but that can bestow upon you some remarkable benefits in the years to come. To keep you loose and centered, we've created a simple routine called the Whole Body Balance and Stretch, covered in the next chapter.

This program won't eat up hours of your day, and you won't need any special equipment or training. But it will help you withstand the demands of daily life, releasing you from the aches and pains that can come from sitting too much, and it will help you prevent dozens of diseases. (During the COVID-19 crisis, exercise was even linked to helping people avoid severe cases.) The Whole Body Fitness Plan will help your joints withstand walking the town at night or exploring a city if you travel; get down on the floor, and UP again, when playing with your grandchildren; not be breathless when taking the stairs. It will help you ski or play tennis or golf more competitively while reducing your risk of injury. And study after study[2] shows that it will also help prevent cognitive decline and keep your brain sharp. Exercise also has positive effects on our microbiome.[3]

Plus, some studies link exercise, particularly high intensity interval training, to increased cellular activity. More muscle + less inflammation + more cellular activity = a healthier metabolism. You may not be able to "boost" your metabolism, but exercise can pre-

Dozens of Reasons to Exercise

Don't be a sitting duck. Inactivity is a primary contributor to dozens of conditions, according to the American Physiological Society. The dangers include:

1. Accelerated aging and premature death
2. Low cardiorespiratory fitness
3. Accelerated sarcopenia
4. Metabolic syndrome
5. Obesity
6. Insulin resistance
7. Prediabetes
8. Type 2 diabetes
9. Nonalcoholic fatty liver disease
10. Coronary heart disease
11. Peripheral artery disease
12. Hypertension
13. Stroke
14. Congestive heart failure
15. Endothelial dysfunction
16. Arterial dyslipidemia
17. Hemostatis
18. Deep vein thrombosis
19. Cognitive dysfunction
20. Depression and anxiety
21. Osteoporosis
22. Osteoarthritis
23. Balance issues
24. Bone fractures and falls
25. Rheumatoid arthritis
26. Colon cancer
27. Breast cancer
28. Endometrial cancer
29. Polycystic ovary syndrome
30. Erectile dysfunction
31. Pain
32. Diverticulitis
33. Constipation
34. Gallbladder disease

vent it from slowing even further with age—and hence, help prevent illness and age-related weight gain.

With the Whole Body Fitness Plan, as you get stronger, fitter, and more mobile, you will FEEL better in and about your body. And beyond that you will feel more energized and happier! That is a lot of return for a just 30 minutes of exercise each day.

Besides, if you weren't at least willing to entertain the idea of changing your daily routine, you would have already skipped over this chapter, and you'd be otherwise occupied exploring some of those delicious recipes toward the end of the book.

But you didn't skip over this chapter. You're here. You're game. And that's great.

Now, all you need is a plan. You'll find that in the next chapter.

— ACTION STEP #11 —

Why exercise? Because it will help you achieve the goals you've set for your future—whether those goals include traveling the world, taking up a new sport, or simply keeping up with current or future grandkids. Exercise is the ultimate expression of optimism.

So let's lay out exactly why you should change into your gym shorts right now. List three goals you have that require you to be healthy and mobile:

1. _____

2. _____

3. _____

Chapter 12

Your Whole Body Fitness Plan

The No-Equipment, No-Excuses Plan to Take Your Strength and Stamina to a Whole New Level

Okay, rock star, let's go and get this! You're at an age where you've earned the right to carve out half an hour a day for yourself. And here's what you're going to do with it: You're going to take care of your body and mind through exercise. And you're going to come away feeling good—because moving your body is how you had fun as a kid, and the more you play as an adult, the more you're going to feel like a kid again.

What you're not going to do, however, is worry about getting it exactly right. Every marathon starts with a first step. What matters right now is that you get into the habit of carving out time. Start with something easy, light, and fun, and take the first week or two to establish your exercise time of the day. Then you can focus on quality and intensity.

Before we begin, though: The workouts in this chapter range from relatively easy to really quite challenging, particularly the high intensity interval training section. Check with your doctor before begin-

Your Magic Muscles

Strongest: Your jaw muscle, or masseter. The Guinness World Record for the strongest bite, set by a Florida man, was 975 pounds.

Fastest: The eyelid muscle, or orbicularis oculi. A blink of an eye, measured by researchers, lasts about 0.3 seconds.

Biggest: The butt muscle, or gluteus maximus. While we're back here, a tushy fat fact: Researchers suggest butt fat may boost cognitive performance because it tends to be higher in brain-boosting omega-3 fatty acids, while belly fat is higher in brain-inhibiting inflammatory compounds. Twerk it!

ning any fitness regime. That goes doubly so if you have significant mobility or cardiac health issues. Outline your plan for your doctor, and ask whether it's appropriate for your current health status—and what you need to do to ensure you'll get the most benefit from exercise with the least amount of worry.

The Essentials of Strength/Resistance, Cardio, and High Intensity Interval Training (HIIT)

Each part of the Whole Body Fitness Plan brings its own benefits. Mixing them together provides even more:

- Cutting down on overuse injuries that can happen when doing longer repetitive movement often
- Pushing you to elevated levels of fitness
- Burning stored carbohydrates, fats, and oxygen, to create overall better metabolic health
- Keeping your interest level high and avoiding burnout

Try a variety of movement throughout the week. Varying your workouts, says Polly de Mille, director of Performance Services at the Hospital for Special Surgery in New York, is like varying your meals. Perhaps one day go on a long bike ride, another a walk in the woods; one day HIIT, and another day swim. Aim for at least two days of strength training. Sports like tai chi and other martial arts are also great ways for people who haven't been active in a while to improve their strength, balance, and flexibility.

Strength/Resistance Training

If we told you that you could be stronger today than you've ever been in your life—even if you're in your fifties or beyond—would you believe us?

Maybe not. After all, we've been taught to think that a slow and steady decline is part of growing older. But it doesn't have to be that way. We're surrounded by examples of people in their fifties and beyond who are in peak physical condition, from Halle Berry to Amazon founder Jeff Bezos to Shark Tank celeb and real estate mogul Barbara Corcoran, thanks to their embrace of fitness and muscle maintenance. "Strength training is paramount to keeping your biological age younger than your chronological age," says Brad Schoenfeld, PhD, associate professor of exercise science at City University of New York Lehman College. The key is to know your own body, understand where you're starting from, and work forward from that point.

Strength/resistance training is simply the practice of putting additional strain, or "resistance," on your muscles. When our muscles meet resistance, our muscle fibers respond by getting stronger and, in the process, helping to keep our bones and muscles strong and to slash our risk of a number of diseases. (We discussed in Chapter 6 how muscle protects against heart disease, stroke, diabetes, cancer, infectious diseases, and pretty much anything else that's out to get you.)

185

If your first thought about strength training is that you don't have a gym membership, feel uncomfortable lifting weights, and dislike the sound of overgrown men grunting like hogs at a trough, don't worry. You never need to walk into a weight room or even pick up a heavy object to do resistance training.

"Resistance training can utilize body weight, dumbbells, kettlebells, resistance bands, laundry soap containers, cans of soup, even cast-iron frying pans," Mark Nutting, certified personal trainer and co-owner of Jiva Fitness in Easton, Pennsylvania, told me. Yoga and Pilates are both forms of resistance training because they call on us to put strain on our muscles, lengthening and strengthening them. Even some forms of endurance exercise, such as calisthenics, mountain biking, rowing, and stair climbing—anything that challenges your muscles—may incorporate resistance training.

You'll know you're getting strong when your body becomes capable of doing more than it could do before—the key term is *progression*. What's important is that you become capable of doing more in the near future. Keep challenging yourself, either with heavier weights or more repetitions (this is known as progressive resistance training, or PRT, because you're "progressively" getting stronger), or by mixing up your workout with new and different exercises.

Cardio Training

Cardio—short for "cardiovascular" and also known as aerobic ("with oxygen")—means any form of exercise that puts a prolonged demand on your heart and lungs. Walking briskly, running a 5K, swimming, biking, dancing, exercising on a machine such as an elliptical trainer, stair climber, or rowing machine—they all qualify as cardiovascular training.

As your heart rate increases to meet the demands of the activity, you pump more blood and oxygen throughout your system. In response to this training, your heart gets stronger and more efficient.

It is able to pump more blood with each heartbeat[1] and you can do more and more activity without it feeling like it is difficult . . . like taking the stairs without being out of breath. Cardiovascular activity lowers resting blood pressure, strengthens blood vessels, lowers bad cholesterol, and improves blood sugar regulation. Your heart and lung system becomes stronger, as does your immune system.[2]

Since the hallmark of a cardio workout includes moving intensely enough to get your heart rate higher than your resting level, you can see that a gentle stroll around the local park doesn't quite cut it. While walking is absolutely a healthy activity that we should all do more of (including those of us who are going to the gym every day), it doesn't count as a cardio workout unless your heart rate and breathing rate rise. When you push yourself enough to feel that increase in breathing, you're getting an aerobic workout. So, up that gentle walk to a brisk walk, take steps, climb a hill if your knees and back allow, intersperse a jog, any which way to increase your heart rate so that you adapt and get stronger and fitter. That is exactly what "training" is. You are training your body to be able to do more, and you will have a greater capacity.

High Intensity Interval Training (HIIT)

HIIT is a workout that combines periods of slow, steady exercise with short bursts of fast, intense exercise. Because it can be both a cardio workout and a strength/resistance workout at the same time, interval training can give you the greatest bang for your buck—maximizing the benefits in less time than it would take to complete two separate workouts.

HIIT intersperses periods of all-out effort (think sprinting) with longer periods of lower-intensity effort. HIIT seems to be particularly effective, especially for older people, but it can be a challenge if you're not used to regular exercise. That said, remember that "high intensity" and "sprinting" mean something different to Usain Bolt

Warming Up to Work Out

When we talk about warming up, we don't mean a long, slow slog on the treadmill. We just mean a few easy, breezy moves that experts call *dynamic motion*. These very simple exercises involve moving our bodies across a range of motion for a period of 60 to 90 seconds each; chances are, you've done a lot of these movements pretty regularly in the past. These warm-ups are also great whenever you want to shake loose the physical stress or mental cobwebs.

Leg Swing: With one hand holding on to a table or wall for balance, swing one leg, within your comfort zone, backward, forward, and across your body side to side. You don't need to go high, just within your comfort zone. Repeat with the opposite leg.

Arm Circles: Stretch your arms out to the sides and draw circles in the air with your hands. The circles don't need to be wide. You're just warming up.

Arm Swings: Stretch your arms out to the sides and then, keeping them straight, swing left across your body, and then back out to your sides. Now stretch right, and then back facing forward.

Lunge: Standing with your feet hip-width apart, take a big step forward with one foot. Lower your hips to feel a bit of a stretch on the top of your forward leg. Then push back up to a standing position. Repeat with the opposite leg.

Lower Back Twist: Stand with your feet hip-width apart and your hands on your hips. Slowly twist your torso as far as you can to one side, keeping your feet flat on the floor, then twist back to the opposite side.

Cat Stretch: Get on the floor on all fours, hands shoulder-width apart, hips over your knees. Arch your back up and hollow out your stomach and hold for a second. Then lower your back and belly toward the floor and hold for a second.

than they do to you: You don't need to charge all-out; you just need to work a little bit harder for brief periods of time.

We'll go deeper into HIIT a little later in this chapter, and even prepare you for it. But first, let's start getting ready to get fit.

Tom Brady, stand aside.

The Whole Body Strength/ Resistance Workout

Do the Whole Body Strength/Resistance Workout two to three times a week—not more, because your body needs time to recover between sessions. Warm up before—see the previous page—and take five to ten minutes after for the Whole Body Balance and Stretch, see page 209.

Each of the workouts consists of a series of isolated exercises—meaning it targets just one muscle (example: a leg extension)—and compound exercises—meaning they involve more than one muscle and joint (example: a squat). Isolated exercises are easier to master and great for beginners, while compound exercises are more efficient because they exercise several muscles at the same time.

"Start first by focusing on making sure your form is correct," says Nutting. Be sure you can follow the motion exactly as it's explained, without pain. If an exercise calls for weights, first try it without weights to make sure you have the range of motion needed. Nutting helped create the workout progression below.

For beginner and intermediate weight training, the best recipe for strength is to do one to three sets of eight to twelve repetitions, according to the American College of Sports Medicine. It can be sets of the same exercise (that's the simplest way), or one set each of three different exercises targeting the same muscle group.

To start, pick the workout below that best describes your current exercise level: Beginner, Intermediate, or Advanced.

- **Beginner:** You have a primarily sedentary lifestyle and don't engage in any sort of strenuous activity more than once a week or so.

- **Intermediate:** You have an active lifestyle but seldom engage in activities that involve lifting, throwing, or jogging.

- **Advanced:** You actively exercise or play sports several times a week and are familiar with basic calisthenics and weight training.

At each level, start with one set of each exercise eight times. Once you're comfortable with eight repetitions and feel no pain (especially in joints like your shoulders and hips), try increasing your repetitions to twelve.

Once that feels comfortable, aim to do two sets of each exercise eight times. Then progress to two sets of twelve repetitions.

Once you're comfortable with that, move to three sets of each exercise eight times. Then progress to three sets of twelve.

When you've mastered this, you can do one of two things: If you really like the workout, try increasing the amount of weight you're lifting. Go back to doing three sets of eight repetitions, and then work your way up to three sets of twelve repetitions. Mastered that? Up the weights again.

If you're ready to try something different, you can move on to the next level.

When you feel confident doing the Advanced workout three times a week, it's time to continue your progression. That may mean consulting a personal trainer, joining a gym, or checking out the many resources available online and in bookstores to help you advance your fitness goals.

BEGINNER

Hup 2–3: Spend five minutes marching in place. To engage both your upper and lower body, alternate reaching one hand and then

What You'll Need

Many of these exercises call for weights, but you don't need to purchase any sort of equipment for this program. While an inexpensive set of light dumbbells is best, if you don't have free weights, just substitute:

- A clean plastic milk jug filled with water or sand (the more you fill it, the heavier it will be)
- Cans of vegetables, beans, or soup that you can comfortably grasp; increase the weight by putting a few cans in a paper or plastic bag with a handle
- A bag of rice or pet food
- A jug of laundry detergent
- A heavy book
- A plastic bottle of soda or juice

How much weight should you lift? Start low—even one or two pounds is fine, especially if you've never lifted before. You know you're in the right range when the final repetition of your final set feels difficult but not impossible. As you get stronger, you can increase the weight, but only as long as you can maintain proper form. Once you surpass the Advanced level, you may want to invest in free weights.

You'll also want a towel, blanket, or mat for the floor exercises.

the other over your head and reaching one hand and then the other across your body. As you warm up, lift your knees higher, allow your marching to become more pronounced.

Chair Squats: Place a chair with its back against a wall for stability. Stand with your back to the chair, your feet shoulder-width apart. Extend both arms out in front of you at shoulder height. Now sit down onto the chair, arms outstretched in front of you for balance, and immediately stand by pushing your feet into the floor and engaging the muscles of your butt and thighs. As you get stronger, make the exercise more challenging by holding a weight with both hands across your chest.

As we age, squats can become crucial for independence, since the glutes and muscles of the upper leg comprise a large amount of muscle in our body.

Row: Place a chair with its back against a wall for stability. Stand facing the chair, feet shoulder-width apart, close enough to the chair so that you can easily reach down and touch the seat. Hold a weight in your right hand, and let your arms hang straight down, so your hands are even with your hips, palms facing your body. Bend forward at the waist with a flat back, your back parallel to the floor, and place your left hand, arm extended, on the seat of the chair for support. Keeping your back parallel to the floor, allow your right arm to extend toward the floor. Now, keeping your right arm close to your side, bend your right elbow, using the muscles of your upper back to pull the weight up until it's next to your rib cage. Slowly lower the weight back to the starting position. Repeat. After eight reps, switch the weight to your left hand and perform the exercise on your left side.

Overhead Press: Stand with your feet hip-width or slightly wider apart with a slight bend in your knees. Do not arch your back. Bring your arms straight in front of you up to your shoulders, bending your elbows so your upper arms are parallel to the floor, elbows at 90 degrees, slightly in front of your ear line, and turn your palms to face forward. Now press one arm up into the air over your head; try to extend your arm fully with just a slight give in the elbow; do not lock your elbow joint. Remain firm in your stance without tipping to the opposite side. Return to the starting position and repeat with the other arm. Once you can complete this motion comfortably, hold a weight in each hand and alternate overhead presses.

Floor Press: Lie on your back, knees bent, feet flat, arms at your side with a weight in each hand. Bend your elbows so your forearms are perpendicular to the floor, palms facing toward your feet. Now, keeping your back straight and your head and shoulders on the floor, use the muscles of your chest and arms to press the weight upward until your arms are straight above. Pause for a moment, then return to the starting position.

Breathe

Exhale as you make the effort (lift, push, or pull) and inhale as you release.

Hip Bridge: Lie on your back, knees bent, feet flat. Rest your arms flat at your sides, palms facing down. Keeping your shoulders, head, and feet on the floor, push up with your hips to raise your butt off the floor; try to create a straight line along your body from your shoulders to your knees. Pause for a moment, then return to the starting position.

Modified Plank: Get on all fours on the floor. Place your knees under your hips and your hands under your shoulders. Bend your elbows and lower yourself to place your forearms flat on the floor, palms down, and keep your shoulders back so your chest doesn't curl inward. Now slowly shift your knees back so that your knees, hips, and shoulders make a straight line. (Your knees remain on the floor.) Engage your abdominals, tightening them and pulling your belly button up toward your spine, and squeeze your butt muscles, pushing your hips toward the floor so that there is no arch in your back. Breathe as you hold the position, building up from 5 to 30 seconds.

Farmer's Walk: Brace your abdominal muscles, and pick up a weight in each hand. Stand with your arms straight down at your sides, palms facing your hips. Stand tall and straight: Pull your shoulders back, and imagine a string at the very top of your head pulling you toward the ceiling. Now, keeping the weights at your sides, walk for 15 seconds. Pause to rest, then repeat.

Back Extension: Lie facedown, forehead resting on the floor, legs straight, toes touching the floor. Bend your elbows and rest your palms on the floor next to your ribs. Now, keeping your neck and back straight, lift your head and shoulders off the floor using the muscles of your back, not your arms, to push yourself up. Hold for three breaths, then lower yourself again to the floor.

As you get stronger, try these progressions:

❑ Extend your arms out to the sides like an airplane; lift up your arms and torso.

❑ With your hands behind your head, elbows wide, lift your head and shoulders up.

❑ With your arms stretched overhead on the floor, palms facing each other, thumbs pointing up, lift your head and shoulders up, then slowly lift your right arm as high as it can go. Then, keeping your head and shoulders up off the floor, lower your right arm and lift your left. Slowly alternate sides.

❑ Lift your shoulders, arms, and legs off the floor all at the same time; push your pubis down into the floor as you and lengthen and extend your legs.

This exercise helps keep our posture and spine strong and counter-

acts the forward motion many of us engage in much of the day sitting in front of screens.

Bird Dog: Get on all fours on the floor, back flat, knees under your hips, and your hands under your shoulders. Tighten your abdominal muscles to keep your back straight and pull your shoulder blades together, as though you were pinching a pencil between them. Now, keeping your back parallel to the floor, lift and extend both your left arm and right knee out as far as you can, as if you were reaching for the front wall with your arm and back wall with your foot while maintaining your balance. Hold for a beat, then return to the starting position. Now lift your right arm and left knee, extend both out, hold for a beat, then return to the starting position.

At first you may have difficulty maintaining your balance as you move. That is the point! You will become more stable as you strengthen your core.

Calf Raise on Steps: Stand on the bottom stair of a staircase, with both heels dangling off the step, your weight on your toes. Hold on to a railing for support. Lower your heels so they are below the level of the stair, then flex your calves to raise up onto your tippy-toes.

As you get stronger, try doing this exercise one leg at a time, with eight reps for each leg.

INTERMEDIATE

Chair Squats with Weight: Place a chair with its back against a wall for stability. Stand with your back to the chair, your feet shoulder-width apart. Hold a light weight in both hands against your chest. Now sit down onto the chair and immediately stand by pushing your feet into the floor and engaging the muscles of your butt and thighs.

Row: Place a chair with its back against a wall for stability. Stand facing the chair, feet shoulder-width apart, close enough to the chair so that you can easily reach down and touch the seat. Hold a weight in your right hand, and let your arms hang straight down, so your hands are even with your hips, palms facing your body. Bend forward at the waist with a flat back, your back parallel to the ground, and place your left hand, arm extended, on the seat of the chair for support. Keeping your back parallel to the ground, allow your right arm to extend toward the floor. Now, keeping your right arm close to your side, bend your right elbow, using the muscles of your upper back to pull the weight up until it's next to your ribcage. Slowly lower the weight back to the starting position. After 8 reps, switch the weight to your left hand and perform the exercise on your left side.

Overhead Press: Place a chair with its back against a wall for stability. Sit in the chair with your back straight, feet flat on the floor. Hold a weight in each hand. Bend and lift your elbows in front of you so your upper arms are parallel to the floor, elbows at 90 degrees, your hands by your ears, palms facing out. Now press your arms up into the air over your head; try to extend your arms fully and touch the two weights together over your head.

Knee Push-ups: Get on all fours on the floor, with your hands at chest level, slightly wider than your body. Keep your elbows in toward your body. Lift your feet so they are off the floor, and lean your weight forward, so your hands are supporting your upper body. Now bend your elbows and lower your chest until it is almost at the floor, then push back up to the starting position.

Hip Bridge: Lie on your back, knees bent, feet flat on the floor close to your butt. Rest your arms flat at your sides, palms down. Keeping your shoulders, head, and feet on the floor, push up with your hips through your heels to raise your butt off the floor; try to create a straight line along your body from your shoulders to your knees. Pause for a moment, then return to the starting position.

Plank: Lie facedown, legs straight, toes touching the floor. Bend your arms at the elbow and rest your forearms on the floor. Now, keeping your neck and back straight, lift your hips and chest off the floor, so your weight is resting on your forearms and toes. Hold for three breaths—or more, as you get stronger—and then lower yourself back to the floor.

Farmer's Walk: Stand tall and straight with your arms down at your sides, weights in each hand, palms facing your hips. Pull your shoulders back and brace your abdominal muscles. Imagine a string at the very top of your head pulling you toward the ceiling. Now, keeping the weights at your sides, walk for 15 seconds. Pause to rest, then repeat.

Superman: Lie facedown, legs straight, toes touching the floor. Extend your arms straight out beyond your head. Now, keeping your neck and back straight, use your back muscles to lift your arms, head, and shoulders off the floor. Hold for three breaths, then lower yourself back to the floor. As you get stronger, you can lift your legs off the floor at the same time you lift your shoulders.

Bird Dog: Get on all fours on the floor, back flat, knees under your hips, and your hands under your shoulders. Tighten your abdominal muscles to keep your back straight and pull your shoulder blades together, as though you were pinching a pencil between them. Now, keeping your back parallel to the floor, lift and extend both your left arm and right knee out as far as you can, as if you were reaching for the front wall with your arm and back wall with your foot while maintaining your balance. Hold for a beat, then return to the starting position. Now lift your right arm and left knee, extend both out, hold for a beat, then return to the starting position.

Step-ups: Stand at the bottom of a staircase, feet hip-width apart and toes pointing forward, holding the railing for support. (You can also use a stable platform.) Now step with your left leg onto the bottom stair and, without pushing off from your back leg, use your left leg to lift your body up. Your left foot should be fully on the step and your hip, knee, and ankle should all be aligned, your knee over your toe; don't lean in toward your body line. Allow your right leg to comfortably dangle behind you. Pause for a moment, then lower your right leg to the floor slowly and return to the starting position. Repeat the movement, this time stepping up with your right leg and keeping your left leg behind you. Pause for a moment, then return to the starting position. As you get stronger, you can go to a higher step and hold weights in your hands, elbows bent so the weights are at shoulder height.

ADVANCED

Air Squats: Stand with your feet shoulder-width apart, feet flat on the floor. Extend both arms in front of you at shoulder height. Now slowly bend your knees and lower your butt as if you were sitting on a chair. When your thighs are parallel to the floor, stop, pause for a moment, and then use your core, gluts, hamstrings, and quads to stand back up a bit more quickly than you squatted down.

Don't squat below parallel or let your knees drift out in front of your toes or inward toward the midline of your body, which can put you at risk for knee problems.

Row: Place a chair with its back against a wall for stability. Stand facing the chair, feet shoulder-width apart. Hold a weight in your right hand. Bend forward at the waist with a flat back (your back should be parallel to the floor) and place your left hand, arm extended, on the seat of the chair for support. Keeping your back parallel to the floor, allow your right arm to extend toward the floor while your right hand is holding a weight. Your palm should be facing your body. Now, keeping your right arm close to your side, bend your right elbow, using the muscles of your upper back to pull the weight up until it's next to your rib cage. Slowly lower the weight back to the starting position. After eight reps, switch the weight to your left hand and perform the exercise on your left side.

Overhead Press: Stand with your back straight, feet flat on the floor, knees slightly bent. Hold a light weight (such as a bottle or can) in each hand. Bend and lift your elbows so your upper arms are parallel to the floor, elbows at 90 degrees, your hands by your ears, palms facing out. Now press your arms up into the air over your head; try to extend your arms fully and touch your hands over your head.

Push-ups: Lie facedown with your legs straight, toes touching the floor, and elbows bent. Place your hands, palms down, on the floor at the sides of your chest. Tighten your abdominal muscles to stabilize your back. Now push up with your palms to raise your chest and abdomen off the floor until your arms are straight; your body should form a straight line from your ankles to your head. Pause for a second, then lower your body until your chest is an inch above the floor. Pause again and push back up.

This exercise can be challenging even for relatively fit people. If you have difficulty with it, consider swapping in Knee Push-ups from the Intermediate workout or combining both types of push-ups throughout the workout.

One-Legged Hip Bridge: Lie on your back with your left leg straight and your right knee bent, right foot flat on the floor, close to your butt. Rest your arms at your sides, palms facing down. Keeping your shoulders, head, and feet on the floor, push up through your right heel to raise your butt and left leg off the floor; your body should form a straight line from your shoulders to your knees and on through to your left foot. Pause for a moment, then return to the starting position. Change legs, so your right leg is straight and your left leg is bent, left foot close to your butt, and repeat the motion.

Plank: Lie facedown, legs straight, toes touching the floor. Bend your arms at the elbow and rest your forearms on the floor below you. Now, keeping your neck and back straight, lift your hips and chest off the floor, so your weight is resting on your forearms and toes. Hold for three breaths—or more, as you grow stronger—then lower yourself back to the floor.

Farmer's Walk: Stand tall and straight with your arms straight down at your sides, weights in each hand, palms facing your hips. Pull your shoulders back and brace your abdominal muscles. Imagine a string at the very top of your head pulling you toward the ceiling. Now, keeping the weights at your sides, walk for 15 seconds. Pause to rest, then repeat.

Superman with Legs Raised: Lie facedown, legs straight, toes touching the floor. Extend your arms straight out beyond your head. Now, keeping your neck and back straight, lift your arms, head, shoulders, and knees so only your lower abdomen and hips are touching the floor. Hold for three breaths—or more, as you grow stronger—then lower yourself back to the floor.

Bird Dog: Get on all fours on the floor, back flat, knees under your hips, and your hands under your shoulders. Tighten your abdominal muscles to keep your back straight, and pull your shoulder blades together, as though you were pinching a pencil between them. Now, keeping your back parallel to the floor, lift and extend both your left arm and right knee out as far as you can, as if you were reaching for the front wall with your arm and back wall with your foot while maintaining your balance. Hold for a beat, then return to the starting position. Now lift your right arm and left knee, extend both out, hold for a beat, then return to the starting position.

Weighted Step-ups: Stand at the bottom of a staircase, holding the railing with your right hand for support. (You can also use a sta-

---

What About Core Training?

Your core refers to the muscles surrounding your lower torso, including your abs as well as the muscles of your lower back and hips. These muscles keep you balanced; protect you from falls, back pain, and injury; and make it possible to perform everyday movements like bending, twisting, lifting, and reaching overhead.

That's why we incorporate squats and the farmer's walk—which fitness professionals say are the two most effective core exercises you can perform—as a regular part of the Whole Body Fitness Plan, in addition to other core exercises for the stomach and lower back.

---

ble platform, if you don't need a railing for support.) With your left hand, hold a weight, allowing it to hang down at thigh level. Now step with your left leg onto the bottom stair and lift your body up as you bend your right leg comfortably behind you. Pause for a moment, then lower your right leg to the floor and return to the starting position. Switch the weight to your right hand, and repeat the movement, this time stepping up with your right leg, keeping your left leg behind you, and using your left hand to hold the railing for support. Pause for a moment, then return to the starting position. As you get stronger, choose a higher step.

The Whole Body Cardio Plan

Do the Whole Body Cardio Workout two to three times a week (or more if you prefer). Warm up before, and take three to ten minutes to cool down afterward by slowing your pace until your heart rate and blood pressure return to normal. Then take five to ten minutes after for the Whole Body Balance and Stretch.

As we said previously, any form of exercise that raises your heart rate and breathing rate qualifies as a cardio workout. Jogging? Cardio workout. Trail hiking? Cardio workout. Dance party? Cardio workout. Gettin' jiggy wit' it? Cardio workout. And if you can get 150 minutes of that a week, we salute you!

The explosion in online classes (check out YouTube), apps, and social media resources has made access to home cardio workouts easier than ever. Many gyms also offer remote classes, and some towns and organizations offer remote classes free. You could probably string together a series of TikTok dances and have yourself a fine cardio workout.

While you're looking to do a cardio workout two to three times a week, if you want more, go for it. Strength/resistance training requires you to rest your muscles for a day after each workout to see maximum results, but you can do cardio six days a week if you'd like.

What's great is that we've built this plan with an eye toward maximum flexibility. Whatever your chosen activity, you can do it in a way that helps your body get progressively fitter.

BEGINNER

Start here if you do not currently engage in any sort of cardiovascular fitness activity.

Work up to 20 to 30 minutes of walking briskly, riding a bike, swimming, participating in an easy dance class, or enjoying any other aerobic activity at a pace where your breathing is easy and you can still talk comfortably. Once you reach a point where 30 minutes of exercise at this level becomes comfortable, progress to Intermediate.

INTERMEDIATE

You're at the intermediate level if you can comfortably walk briskly, ride a bike, swim, or engage in other cardiovascular fitness activity for 30 minutes at a time, at least twice a week.

Work up to 30 to 40 minutes of brisk walking, easy running, moderately intense bike riding, exercising using a machine, or enjoying any other aerobic activity at a pace where your breathing is lightly labored—you can still carry on a conversation, but it is challenging. Once you reach a point where 30 to 40 minutes at this pace becomes comfortable, progress to Advanced.

ADVANCED

You are at the advanced level if you can comfortably run, hike, or bike briskly, take spin or aerobics classes, or engage in other demanding cardiovascular fitness activity for at least 30 minutes at a time, and if you do so at least twice a week.

First, congratulations: You have a solid foundation in cardiovascular fitness. Keep up the good work! To up your game even more, consider integrating high intensity interval training (HIIT) into your weekly workouts. You'll read more about HIIT below.

The Whole Body High Intensity Interval Workout

Research shows that just ten minutes of high intensity interval training—exercise that combines brief periods of intense work with longer periods of easier exercise—can have a dramatic impact. And for people just starting HIIT, it may take as little as one minute of hard work three times a week to see marked improvements.

And here's the crazy part: This plan has been shown to work better on older bodies than it does on teenagers.

You can apply this approach to any kind of exercise. If you're a runner, swimmer, hiker, cycler, or walker, HIIT can be part of your workout. And you can apply HIIT to weight training, calisthenics, even Pilates. We'll walk you through strength/resistance and cardio HIIT workouts here.

How Can I Get Myself to Actually Do the Workouts?

We humans are incredibly skilled at self-sabotage. You never read about squirrels going, "Store up nuts for the winter? Nah . . ." They just follow their instincts. But we tend to overthink everything, and that can lead us to not doing what we should to take care of ourselves.

The good news is that once you get into the habit of fitness, it's a lot easier to stick with it. A review of studies in the *British Journal of General Practice* found that it took about ten weeks to form new habits and make them seem automatic. Here, then, are some tricks to help you rack up a solid string of workouts:

Find a partner. "It holds you accountable, because you don't want to let them down by not showing up, and you'll also have more fun," says Deborah Feltz, professor of kinesiology at Michigan State University. In her research, Feltz has found other benefits, too: People who work out with a partner exert more effort and spend almost twice as much time exercising as those who go it alone. And your partner doesn't even need to be by your side; even a virtual partner exercising along with you remotely could help boost your results.

Do something you enjoy. Exercise doesn't have to mean sweating in the gym or endless treadmill time. How about hiking a local greenway, taking a dance class, or volunteering to walk dogs at the local animal shelter? If you choose an activity you genuinely like, research shows you're much more inclined to stick with it over time.

Prioritize convenience. One study found that the shorter the distance to the gym, the more likely members were to go. Another shows that people who live in neighborhoods with sidewalks are 47 percent more likely to be active for at least 39 minutes a day than residents of areas without sidewalks. "Set your workout clothes next to your bed the night before, and keep exercise equipment visible and nearby," says David Maxfield, coauthor of *Change Anything: The New Science of Personal Success*. "If you have a treadmill or exercise bike on the first floor, you're twice as likely to use it than if it's in the basement."

Reward yourself. Some studies have found that people who establish rewards or other incentives for working out are more likely to stick to their exercise programs. And, when those rewards are taken away, they're typically more likely to fall off their programs as well. Here are some ideas on how to put this concept to work:

- **Find a challenge.** Training for a 5K or a charity bike ride is a great way to keep yourself motivated and focused. Most events offer at least a T-shirt for participating, which you'll get to wear while working out as a constant reminder of your accomplishment. And it's cool to tell others that you're training for something special, rather than just exercising.
- **Pay yourself.** Set a goal of a certain number of workouts each week. If you stick to it for a month, buy yourself a gift. Or stick two bucks in a jar for each workout and splurge at the end of the month with your savings.
- **Or fine yourself.** Negative reinforcement can work, too. Charge yourself $5 each time you skip a workout, and give the money to a charity at the end of the month. Or consider betting a friend or co-worker that you'll stick to your program. If you slack off, they win and you lose.

Keep a workout diary. If you don't track your progress digitally, try keeping a written diary of what you've accomplished week by week. We tend to underestimate our own personal achievements; make sure you have written testimony on how far you've come.

HIIT may offer benefits beyond fitness. A 2018 study found that higher-intensity workouts may blunt immune system decline in older adults[3] as well. And that's not all. HIIT can also:

Recharge your cells. Researchers at the Mayo Clinic found that people ages sixty-five to eighty who incorporated HIIT into their walking or biking programs made more proteins for their energy-producing mitochondria, effectively slowing down aging at a cellular level. And the older you are, the greater its impact, according to studies.

Flatten your belly. Another study of sedentary women compared 20 minutes of HIIT with 40 minutes of steady-state exercise. The HIIT subjects were the only ones who lost fat—primarily belly fat.

Protect your heart. In a study of nearly five thousand people with heart disease, researchers found that HIIT did more to protect the subjects from future heart problems than traditional moderate workouts.

Keep you active longer. A Japanese study put 696 people of middle age or older on a walking program that incorporated HIIT workouts. Seventy percent were still doing the workout twenty-two months later.

Boost testosterone. A study of twenty-two sedentary men in their sixties found that regular exercise plus HIIT sprints on a bike increased their testosterone by 17 percent in twelve weeks.

Parts of your brain may also get a greater boost from this type of exercise than from either resistance training or straight cardio. When researchers studied MRIs of people during exercise, they found that low-intensity periods seem to trigger parts of the brain used in cognition and attention, while high-intensity periods activate neurological networks involved in emotional processing.

One caveat: With interval training, it is especially important to do warm-up exercises. If you are doing something with repetitive motion such as walking, running, biking, swimming, or training on the elliptical, you can warm up by starting slow and building up speed. If you are going to do a calisthenics-style, strength-training, mixed-movement HIIT, consult Warming Up to Work Out on page 188.

Is HIIT for You?

Before going for HIIT, make sure you have a foundational fitness level and the mobility to do the moves. Also, even though HIIT is appealing, it may not be for everyone. Some people like the meandering time spent outdoors hiking or cycling through towns, getting lost in the rhythm of movement and taking time to problem solve and think creatively. HIIT is quick and intense and requires a focus on your form and your next step. It can be exhilarating and satisfying to know how hard you worked. Check it out and see what works best for you.

Interval Training: How Much Is Enough?

You may want to do HIIT only once or twice a week as it can take time for you to recover.

HIIT Strength/Resistance Training

Here's an example of how to integrate HIIT and strength/resistance training. Since intensity is key, start with the beginner level, even if you consider yourself already fit. You can use any combination of the resistance exercises in this chapter but try to hit an array of both upper and lower body moves.

	BEGINNER: TOTAL TIME 16 MINUTES	INTERMEDIATE: TOTAL TIME 30 MINUTES	ADVANCED: TOTAL TIME 45 MINUTES
Work Interval	30 seconds	1 minute	1 minute
Rest Interval	30 seconds	30 seconds	15 seconds
Number of exercises	4	5	6
Rounds	4	4	6

HIIT Cardio Training

HIIT workouts can also be applied to cardio. Here are three simple HIIT workouts. They're demanding, so if you haven't done HIIT before, you'll probably want to start at the beginner level.

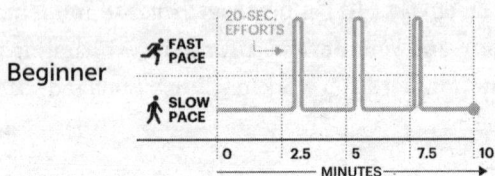

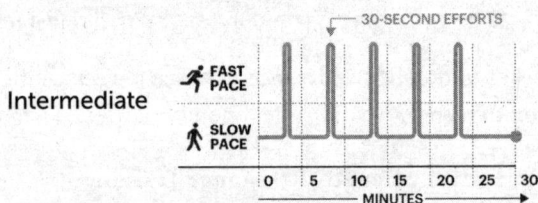

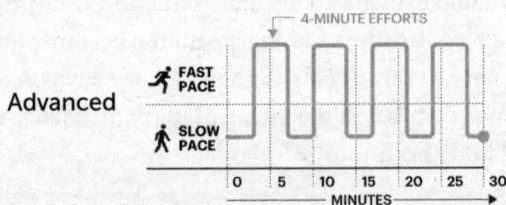

The Whole Body Balance and Stretch

A lot of us labor—literally—under the impression that if we're not working hard and breaking a sweat, we're not really "exercising." But that's not at all true. Two crucial aspects of fitness require little if any huffing and puffing, yet they're essential to our overall well-being: flexibility—achieved through stretching— and balance. Let's take a look at each.[4]

Flexibility Through Stretching

Joint flexibility decreases as we age; shoulder flexibility, in particular, drops about 6 degrees per decade in women, and 5 degrees per decade in men, between the ages of fifty-five and eighty-six. Imagine starting from the point where you can reach both hands straight up into the air and touch them together over your head; as time goes by, your elbows will need to bend more and more to get those hands to touch. But with flexible joints, we can tie our shoes, put on a sweater, and reach that high shelf in the pantry. And flexibility goes hand in hand with strength; tight muscles can't generate the sort of explosive force needed to move quickly and with power. A diminished range of motion can hinder our walking speed and increase our risk of falls. It can also increase our chances of back pain because stiff muscles often don't get enough nutrients, which leads to the development of "trigger points," or sore spots along our spine.

There are two ways to improve flexibility.

The first is dynamic movement, covered in our warm-ups. Prior to each workout, first thing in the morning, or after sitting for long periods of time, try some of those dynamic warm-ups.

The second is static stretching. A static stretch involves holding a stretched position for 30 to 60 seconds. This type of stretching is best done after a cardio, strength/resistance, or HIIT workout, when your muscles are already warmed up. Run through the following series for five to ten minutes.

Here are some to try.

Shoulder Corner Stretch: Stand facing the corner of a room, a little less than arm's length from each wall. Bend both arms at the elbow 45 degrees and press each elbow against a wall. Lean in toward the corner so you feel a stretch across your chest. Hold for 30 to 60 seconds. Relax and repeat.

Standing Quadriceps Stretch: Stand about a foot away from a wall, facing the wall. Rest your left arm against the wall for balance. Bend your right knee and lift your right foot up behind you, so your lower leg is about parallel with the floor. Now, with your right hand, reach down and grab your right foot. Gently pull upward on the foot so you feel a light stretch in the front of your right thigh. Hold for 30 to 60 seconds, then gently release your foot and lower it to the floor. Using your right arm for balance, switch to your left leg. Relax and repeat.

Hip and Thigh Stretch: Stand tall with your feet about two shoulder widths' apart. Turn your feet, hips, and shoulders to the right. Now bend your right leg and lower your body so that your right thigh is parallel with the floor and your right calf is vertical. Lower your body as much as you feel comfortable, until you feel a stretch in the muscles on the inside of your left thigh. Hold for 30 to 60 seconds, then straighten back up to the starting position. Repeat the motion on the left side. Relax and repeat.

Iliotibial Band Stretch: Did you know your body comes with its own band? Two of them, actually, called the iliotibial (ITB) bands. The ITB is a thick band of tissue that runs down the outside of each of your thighs, connecting your hips to your knees. When an ITB gets tight, it can cause hip pain, knee pain, or both. To stretch the

ITBs, sit on the floor with your legs stretched out in front of you and your back straight. Place your hands on the floor next to you for balance. Bend your right knee and place your right foot on the floor on the outside of your left knee. Turn your head and shoulders so you are facing toward the right. Lift your left arm and place it against the outside of your right knee. Now gently press your left arm against your right knee, pushing it farther across your body; you should feel a stretch along the right side of your hip and spine. Hold for 30 to 60 seconds, then repeat on the opposite side. Relax and repeat.

Lying Figure Four: Lie on your back with your knees bent. Cross your right ankle over your left knee and rest it there. Now reach both hands up and grasp your left leg just below the knee. Gently pull your left leg toward you, being sure to keep your upper body flat against the floor. Hold for 30 to 60 seconds. Repeat on the opposite side. Relax and repeat.

Balance

Falls are the second biggest cause of accidental death after traffic injuries, according to the World Health Organization. The Centers for Disease Control reports that more than one in four Americans over sixty-five experiences a fall each year, and falls are the leading cause of head injuries and broken hips. So the time to focus on balance is now, not when you're older and at risk. Don't wait until it starts raining to fix the roof.

Balance is a surprisingly complex function; it requires many different systems in the body to work well together. To balance properly, we need strength, especially in the lower body and core, and flexibility, especially in the hips and lower back.

These become more important as we age because aging presents several other challenges. The vestibular system, a complex system of sensory organs that helps us detect where we are in space, also declines with age, as does our reaction time. Our eyesight, especially our peripheral vision and our ability to detect subtle changes in shadows, diminishes. This is why walking at dusk on an uneven ground can become challenging. Medications may also interfere with stability and balance. In essence, a multitude of control mechanisms all converge to throw us off balance. But we can train for it. We can get stronger and more prepared.

In other words, do not blow off this part of the fitness program. Years from now, your body will thank you.

We recommend adding a few minutes of Stretch and Balance to each workout, simply because you're more likely to remember to do it then. But the truth is, you can do the balance exercises at any time—before, after, or between workouts. They do not require a warm-up. You can even do them at random times within a day, like while waiting in line or online or brushing your teeth! But remember that, like any other type of fitness training, this series of exercises is designed to challenge your body and stimulate your muscles and your brain to adapt and get better. Here's how to do it.

Weight Shifting: Stand upright with your feet hip-width apart. Keep your back straight and tighten your abdominal muscles. Now simply shift weight from one foot to the other. As you do this, keep your abdominals tight; try not to slouch or let your hips tilt toward one side or the other. When you shift your weight, pause and hold, building up to 30 seconds on each side before you shift to the other side.

As you get stronger, try these progressions:

❑ Shift weight onto one leg and bend your other leg, bringing your knee up. Balance on one foot. Repeat on the opposite side.

❑ Stand facing a wall, resting your right hand on the wall for support. Lift your left leg. Remove your right hand from the wall, so that you're balancing on your right foot. Now close your eyes (keeping close to the wall in case you need to reach out for support). Repeat on the opposite side.

Single Leg Dynamic Movement: Stand with your feet hip-width apart, with a wall or table on your right, about a foot away. Shift your weight onto your right foot. Now reach your left leg out to the front, then back to neutral without touching the floor, then to the side, back to neutral and to the back, and back to neutral. If you need to touch your left foot down briefly to restabilize, do so. Don't be shy about grabbing the wall or table for balance if you need it. Now turn around so the wall or table is to your left and perform the same motions with your right leg. As you progress, rotate through a continuous progression of front, side, and back extensions as you stand on one leg, without having to touch the opposite foot down between movements.

March in Place: March in place and as you lift one knee, reach the alternate arm straight overhead (lift your right knee and left arm, then left knee and right arm).

Seesaw: Stand upright with a table or wall at your right, about a foot away. Lift your right knee so your right thigh is parallel to the floor. Bend your elbows at 45 degree angles. Lean forward carefully as you push your right leg back behind you; simultaneously bring your right elbow forward and your left elbow back, mimicking a running motion. Now bring your right leg to the front as your right elbow moves backward and your left elbow moves forward. Reach out to grab the wall or table for extra balance if you need it. Repeat this motion five times, then turn around so that the wall is at your left and repeat the entire exercise with your left leg.

Heel-to-Toe Walk: Stand next to a wall or kitchen counter so that you can touch it to help you balance. Place one foot directly in line and in front of the other so that the heel of your forward foot barely touches the toes of your back foot. Balance this way without moving. Try taking your hand off of the wall or counter. When you feel comfortable, try walking forward slowly, heel to toe, heel to toe. When you reach the end of the counter, turn around and walk back in the heel-to-toe pattern. When that becomes easy, walk backward in a reverse toe-to-heel pattern.

— ACTION STEP #12 —

How many mornings have you woken up with a vague plan to work out, only to go to bed that night having not achieved your goal? It happens to all of us. Sometimes making the transition from stillness to motion can be the hardest part of exercising.

Let's take some steps to overcome the inertia. List three reasons why you're most likely to skip out on a workout. Then, write down something you can do to overcome that obstacle. Some great tips include enlisting a partner, having comfortable workout clothes, scheduling workouts just the way you schedule meetings or lunches, and betting someone that you can fit in a certain number of workouts each week.

My Excuse   **My Strategy to Overcome It**

_____   _____

_____   _____

_____   _____

Chapter 13

Troubleshooting the Whole Body Reset

Frequently Asked Questions and Easily Solved Dilemmas

No one ever got better at a task without facing some challenges. Which is why we could never have created the book you hold in your hands without the input of the more than one hundred AARP employees who joined the Whole Body Reset test panel.

They helped prove just how effective this program is, by dropping an average of five pounds, with one in three losing ten pounds or more in just twelve weeks. But more important, they challenged us with pointed questions that made us think harder, drove us deeper into the research, and helped to ensure that the Whole Body Reset was not just effective, but easy to use as well.

Here are some of the questions our test panel asked—questions that might be relevant to you as well—and some additional ideas that will guide you through the life-changing experience of the Whole Body Reset.

Q: You say right in the introduction that the more diets you go on, the greater your likelihood of gaining weight in the future. Why is the Whole Body Reset safer?

A: Most diets tend to be rigid, with lots of rules that you can really follow only for a certain amount of time. Some cut out whole food groups or make you skip meals at certain times of the day, making socializing a challenge. And worst of all, many diets promise fast weight loss.

Fast weight loss can be bad for you. It can hurt bone health, exacerbate muscle loss, and lead to a slower metabolism and future weight gain. In fact, dieting is a stronger predictor of weight gain than even genetics: In a really interesting study[1] of twins, researchers found that when one of the pair dieted to lose weight, the dieter gained progressively more weight than the nondieting twin.

The Whole Body Reset, on the other hand, isn't a diet you go on and then go off. It's about learning to adopt habits—like eating protein throughout the day, being conscious of fiber intake, making vegetables your friend—that will help you prevent future weight gain. One of the goals is to preserve your metabolism right where it is, and put an end to muscle loss and that creeping one to two pounds per year of weight gain that most of us experience after age fifty. Instead of short-term weight loss, the Whole Body Reset is designed for lifelong health, mobility, and energy.

Q: Is the Whole Body Reset a "low-carb" diet?

A: No. When we say, "focus on protein," a lot of people hear "eat low-carb." But that's a mistake. Nutrient-rich carbohydrates are an important part of any food plan because that's where you'll find many of the vitamins and minerals you need, and all of the fiber as well.

The kinds of carbs we tend to overeat are refined, starchy carbs—the white breads and crackers, cakes and cookies, pastas and grains.

The key, then, is to focus on that critical phrase "nutrient-rich." Whole grains, sweet potatoes, beans—all are starches, but they pack plenty of the vitamins, minerals, and fiber we need.

A good rule of thumb is to eat at least half of your starchy carbs from whole grain foods each day. That means if you eat six to eight servings of starch a day, choose at least four that are unprocessed. That leaves some room for other foods. About 10 percent of your calories (between 150 and 200 calories) can come from "discretionary" calories. Birthdays happen, and so do weddings and date nights, and denying ourselves the foods that come along with these moments isn't good for the soul. So if that sandwich goes best on a ciabatta roll, go for it. If it's bad luck not to have a slice of birthday cake, who are we to tempt the fates? But look for opportunities to balance out the rest of the day by choosing higher fiber foods.

Q: How much do I have to worry about portion size?

A: Have you ever heard the phrase "portion distortion"? It refers to the idea that what we see as a standard serving of food today—typically a serving of starches or sweets such as pasta, bread, or soda—would look enormous to our grandparents. According to the National Institutes of Health, a generation ago the average bagel was 3 inches in diameter; today it's 6 inches. A medium bag of popcorn used to be 5 cups; today it's 11 cups. And a standard soda was 6½ ounces, whereas today it's a whopping 20 ounces!

That makes trying to keep our weight in check even more difficult. While it's possible to overdo it on fruits, vegetables, and meats, we're most likely to overeat refined starches and sweets—all those soft, chewy, crunchy, salty, sugary things we think of as "comfort food." And because those foods are inexpensive to produce, it's exactly where food marketers are most likely to push portion size, to make it seem like we're getting our money's worth.

Remember, what you get served at a restaurant is often much

more than a single serving, so you could be eating *lots* more than you think. A single burrito with rice and beans at Chipotle could have as many as six servings of carbs—three from the tortilla itself, another four if they load up the rice and beans. A handful of gummies is also a serving. The CDC's chart, adapted from the American Diabetes Association, will give you an idea of what a serving of starch looks like. (Go to cdc.gov, and in the search bar, enter "carbohydrate choice list.")

The chart tells us, for example, that one serving of an English muffin is half a muffin; a serving of a baked potato is 3 ounces, or about a quarter of a large potato; a serving of granola is ¼ cup; a serving of baked potato chips is about eight chips.

Q: Getting 25 grams of protein at breakfast is hard—especially since my doctor says not to eat eggs every day. How can I do it?

A: Eggs have about 6 grams of protein each, so they're a solid choice for days when you're having trouble meeting your goal. But there are plenty of other egg-free ways to get to 25 grams or more—often just by adding seeds or nuts to your favorite breakfast foods. Here are a few easy high-protein breakfasts:

- 1 cup cottage cheese (25 g)

- Whey protein smoothie (a scoop of protein powder is usually 20 g or more)

- 2 packets instant oatmeal (8 g) in 1 cup milk (8 g) with 1 oz chopped almonds (5 g), and 2 tbsp hemp seeds (7 g)

- ½ whole wheat bagel (5 g) with 3 oz lox (15 g) and 2 tbsp cream cheese (2 g), plus 1 oz pumpkin seeds (5 g)

- 1 cup plain Greek yogurt (20 g) with 2 tbsp ground flax seeds (3 g), ¼ cup mixed nuts (6g), and berries

- Breakfast burrito with ¾ cup chopped tofu (15 g) scrambled (like an egg!) with 1 oz cheese (5 g) and ½ cup black beans (4.5 g) wrapped in a flour tortilla (1 g)

- 2 tbsp peanut butter (7 g) and a sliced banana (1.5 g) on 2 slices whole wheat bread (8 g), and 1 cup of milk (8 g)

Q: Eating 25 to 30 grams of fiber in a day sounds like a lot. How can I get there without eating salad all day?

A: First of all, salads aren't always the best way to get more fiber. Many people eat a green salad and think, "I'm getting my fiber," but a cup of lettuce provides less than 2 grams of fiber. The key is to pack our diet with fruits and vegetables as well as whole grains, beans, nuts, and other plant foods. Shoot for 5 or more grams at each meal and make sure each snack has 2 grams of fiber as well. Here are a few simple swaps you can make that will make a huge difference in your fiber intake:

- Breakfast: Instead of two slices of white bread toast, eat two slices of whole grain toast—1.4 g vs. 3.8 g
- Breakfast: Instead of butter, eat ¼ avocado—0 g vs. 3.4 g
- Snack: Instead of 5 saltines and cheese, eat an apple and cheese—1 g vs. 4.4 g
- Snack: Instead of a granola bar, eat yogurt and ¾ cup of blueberries—1.3 g vs. 2.7 g
- Lunch: Instead of chicken soup, eat lentil soup—1.5 g vs. 6 g
- Lunch: Instead of a 1-ounce side of chips, eat ⅓ cup of dry roasted peanuts—1.2 g vs. 4 g
- Dinner: Instead of ½ cup of white rice, eat ½ cup brown rice—0.7 g vs. 2 g

TOTAL: 7.1 grams vs. 26.3 grams

Q: Are protein supplements a healthy choice? And if so, what kind should I use?

A: Many experts believe there's a king of all proteins, at least when it comes to people 50+: whey protein.

Whey is a part of milk, the part that's discarded in the process of making most cheeses. In a small study of sixteen men and fifteen women, ages sixty-five to eighty, researchers divided the participants into two groups. One group was given whey protein, while the other was given another form of protein (collagen peptides). After two weeks of restricted activity, the subjects in the whey protein group recovered muscle strength more quickly.

Try mixing whey protein powder with almond or regular milk for a low-calorie, high-protein drink; or use it to thicken a smoothie (with or without yogurt); or add it to oatmeal.

Q: I know the meals are packed with fiber and protein, but it seems like I am eating a lot. Won't I gain weight?

A: Remember that the Whole Body Reset isn't a typical weight-loss program. Its first priorities are to stop age-related weight gain and muscle loss and help you maintain your strength, health, and mobility for life. To that end, it makes sense that you may feel as though you're eating plenty; fiber and protein help you feel full. Many people in our pilot panel felt like they were eating a lot—but they still lost weight.

That said, your body isn't the same as anyone else's. Some of us will need more food; some less. If you want to eat less food, or if you want to turbocharge the weight-loss aspect of the Whole Body Reset, start by paying attention to your starchy carbs and portion sizes. You may even want to measure out your carb servings for a few days, to fully understand how much you're actually eating versus what a serving is. If, for example, you normally eat one cup of cooked rice, you may want to try two-thirds of a cup. Small changes like that can add up to big results over time. That one tweak alone will cut 60 to 100 calories out of your day, which could be enough to spark weight loss.

At least half of the starchy carbs you eat should be from high-fiber, whole-food sources, such as brown rice, sweet potatoes, beans, and oatmeal. See if there are any refined carbs—that is, processed foods—hiding in your day that you can eliminate. And make sure you're eating plenty of nonstarchy vegetables (such as greens, broccoli, cauliflower, and brussels sprouts) to keep up your fiber intake.

If you do find you're gaining weight, you may be overdoing it on healthy but high-calorie fats—such as olive oil, nuts, nut butters, and avocado. Remember to keep portion size in mind as you plan out each meal and snack.

Q: I sometimes find myself eating without thinking—I pick up whatever is around the office. How can I stop instinctively noshing?

A: You've heard the term "mindless eating" before—it's what you do when watching a movie, when your hand hits the bottom of the popcorn bucket before the film's halfway over. Problem is, most of us graze throughout our day, every day—nibbling on snacks because they're there, or continuing to pick at a big serving of food even after our bellies send the all-full signal. Food isn't just about hunger; it's about comfort and emotion and bonhomie.

But if we can bring the idea of mindfulness to our eating habits, we can learn to remove those mindless calories that pile up. Try tuning into these three mindful practices as you eat.

First, recognize how hungry you are before you reach for food. Eating is best when accompanied by a feeling of hunger. See the hunger scale (following) for reference:

1. Starving, weak, dizzy

2. Very hungry, cranky, low energy, lots of stomach growling

3. Pretty hungry, stomach is growling a little

4. Starting to feel a little hungry

5. Satisfied, neither hungry nor full

6. A little full, pleasantly full

7. A little uncomfortable

8. Feeling stuffed

9. Very uncomfortable, stomach hurts

10. So full you feel sick

If you wait until you are starving (1 or 2) to eat, you are more likely to eat until you are stuffed (9 or 10). If you eat when you are moderately hungry (3 or 4), it is easier to stop when you are comfortably satisfied (7 or 8). Be aware of when you're no longer hungry; that is the signal that you have had enough, so get in the habit of paying attention to your body's signals, and stop eating when the time comes.

Second, take time to fully taste your food. Enjoy each bite. Notice the texture, taste, consistency, and even the aroma. Finish each bite before taking the next one. Put your fork down and take a sip of water. We tend to eat too many meals at our desks or in front of a screen, and as a result, we've learned to pay attention to something other than our food. When you truly savor your food, you may find that you actually eat less—and enjoy the food more.

Third, plate your food. Whether it is a meal or a snack, do not eat out of the container or bag. Place your portion on a plate. It helps to visually see what and how much you are eating. You can still have seconds!

Q: I like the idea of keeping a food diary so I know I'm really eating what I think I'm eating. Any suggestions?

A: Consider using a tool like eatracker.com, created by Canadian dieticians, which is pretty intuitive and can give you the nutrition information you need while helping you judge serving sizes. (The USDA discontinued its own version, called Supertracker, in 2018.) Or you can use an app on your phone; check your app store for ratings and reviews. If you prefer paper and pen, the American Heart Association offers a downloadable food tracker that you can print out and fill in.

Q: The Whole Body Reset recommends two to three servings of dairy a day. What are substitutes for people who are lactose intolerant or don't process dairy products well?

A: We love dairy because it provides two nutrients essential to preserving muscle and bone: protein and calcium. It's easy for most people to get protein from other sources, but you may have to pay attention to get the recommended amount of calcium—1,000 milligrams a day for men ages fifty-one to seventy and 1,200 milligrams for men over seventy; 1,200 milligrams for women over fifty. Calcium is important for muscle and bones as well as maintaining a healthy blood pressure. Dairy is also high in the amino acid leucine, which is crucial to stimulating muscle protein synthesis.

If you are lactose intolerant, you may want to experiment with dairy products that are easier on your digestion, such as yogurt, kefir, and aged cheeses. Lactose-free dairy is also an option, as are lactase tablets, which can make traditional dairy foods more tolerable for many people. If you rule out dairy altogether, try these non-dairy choices:

- Canned sardines and salmon with bones
- Soybeans, soy products such as tofu made with calcium sulfate, soy yogurt, and tempeh

- Kidney, white, and navy beans
- Collard greens, turnip greens, mustard greens, kale, and bok choy
- Calcium-fortified juices, cereals, breads, rice milk, and almond milk
- Chia seeds and sesame seeds
- Almonds

It's best to try to get the majority of your calcium needs from food, but to top off your intake, check with your doctor about taking a calcium supplement.

Q: You warn about processed foods, but does it really make a difference if my meals are prepackaged or made from scratch?

A: Consider this: In a recent small study, volunteers were put on a diet of either unprocessed foods (fruits, vegetables, lean meats, and whole grains) or ultraprocessed foods (baked goods, cured meats, and snack foods). Participants were presented with the same amounts of overall calories, protein, and carbohydrates, and allowed to eat as much as they wanted. Then, after fourteen days, the volunteers switched to the other diet.

Researchers found that when presented with ultraprocessed foods, subjects ate an average of 500 calories a day more than when they were given whole foods. They also gained an average of two pounds on the ultraprocessed diet, while losing an average of two pounds on the whole-food diet.

Q: Any tips on preparing food in advance? I'm not a big cooking fan, so the less time I spend in the kitchen, the better.

A: Prepping food in advance is one of the easiest ways to make a healthy diet automatic. If you can spare a couple of hours over the course of a weekend, you can prep nearly everything you need for the week. This is especially helpful if you bring your lunch to work each day.

Start by cooking up some grains. A few cups of quinoa, brown rice, or whole wheat pasta can be cooked and stored in the fridge to provide a base for meals in the coming week. You can also cook up beans or lentils and add spices, so you can just ladle the beans over the grains, stick the plate in the microwave, and press "reheat."

In the oven, roast cauliflower, broccoli, brussels sprouts, and sweet potatoes with some olive oil, sea salt, and fresh thyme or rosemary. These, too, can be stored in the fridge for the coming week.

On the grill or stovetop, grill some chicken breasts as your go-to protein because they're easy to reheat and go with just about everything. Then, on days when you have a bit more time, you can cook a steak or some fish.

Also, make sure you have fresh fruit and a source of dairy you enjoy—cheese, yogurt, cottage cheese, milk—on hand at all times.

And finally, consider some simple store-bought condiments. You can eat your precooked protein, grains, and veggies in their natural state, or you can add BBQ sauce, salsa, tomato sauce, pesto, kimchi, harissa, sofrito, or romesco sauce—all available in jars and cans in your supermarket. Play around with some new flavors to see what tickles your palate.

Q: In emotionally charged times, I often revert to binge eating, which leaves me feeling physically, emotionally, and mentally shattered. How can I break this cycle?

A: We all deal with negative emotions in our own ways, and many times those ways aren't healthy. Emotional eating is a particularly difficult issue, because we live in a world that is constantly sending us a message: If we eat this, right now, we'll feel better. Recent research has suggested a few ways to help quell these cravings:

Talk first. If you're eating to manage difficult emotions, consider reaching out to someone with whom you can share those feelings—someone who won't judge you for wanting to eat to deal with them. Tell yourself you can always eat after the conversation.

Short-circuit the feelings with a physical release. A small 2015 study of overweight people who enjoy sugary snacks found that just 15 minutes of moderate exercise (in this case, brisk walking) significantly reduced cravings for sugary snacks.

Drink more water. We often misinterpret thirst as hunger. If you're craving food, try drinking a large glass of water, and see if the craving doesn't pass in a few minutes.

Q: My husband's cardiologist suggested to him that he switch over to a plant-based diet. Any tips on how to get enough protein without meat?

A: "Plant-based" can mean a number of things; in many cases, it just means eating fewer animal products and more plant-based foods. But it could also mean going completely vegetarian, or even 100 percent vegan. Regardless, there are ways of adapting the Whole Body Reset to your needs.

When eating plants only, it's important to combine foods to get a complete set of proteins, which is critical for maintaining muscle. Quinoa, soy (edamame, tofu, and tempeh), seiten, buckwheat (use it to make pancakes!), pumpkin seeds, hemp seeds, and sprouted grain bread are all sources of complete protein.

Otherwise, a great rule of thumb is to combine whole grains (brown rice, whole wheat bread, oats) with legumes, nuts, and seeds (beans, lentils, peanut and nut butters, chia and sunflower seeds). Top pastas with a protein source like peas, walnuts, or toasted pine nuts for a complete meal, or look for chickpea-, bean-, and soy-based pastas that are even higher in protein than your average wheat brand (and taste great). Soups that combine grains and legumes, like pasta fagioli, or red beans and rice provide complete proteins as well.

Finally, try a plant-based protein powder, and combine it with a milk alternative, half a banana, and some frozen berries for a delicious smoothie. Look for a "complete" protein, meaning one that contains a variety of plant proteins, rather than one derived from a single plant source. In particular, make sure it contains leucine, an amino acid that helps stimulate muscle growth, but is often missing from plant-based foods. You can find plant-based protein powders in any vitamin or health-food store, or online.

Q: I've lost three pounds in five weeks, which isn't a lot, but I do feel better, more energetic, lighter. I'm also a little happier. Is that a side effect?

A: Happiness is potentially a side effect of the Whole Body Reset, especially if you've stepped up your exercise levels. Studies consistently show that exercise is associated with a positive outlook.

In addition, several key Whole Body Reset nutrients have also been linked to a lighter, happier mood. Folate, a B vitamin found in legumes and green vegetables, can help improve levels of the happiness hormone serotonin and has been shown in some studies to be deficient in people with depression. Researchers have also found that depression is less common in parts of the world where people eat a lot of fish, leading researchers to surmise that omega-3 fatty acids found in fish (as well as in flax seeds, chia seeds, and walnuts) may be effective in helping to treat mood disorders.

But it's not just what you *are* eating on the Whole Body Reset. It's also what you are *not* eating. People who eat a lot of fried food, especially fast food, are getting high doses of omega-6 fatty acids, which are found in vegetable oils used in frying. When your ratio of omega-6 to omega-3 rises, your risk of depression may also increase.

And a 2017 study found that men who consumed high amounts of sugar were at greater risk of depression as well.

Want more happiness? Try getting outside more often: In one study, researchers found that twenty minutes in a park boosted well-being.

Q: I don't particularly like fruits or vegetables except for carrots, oranges, and apples. Can I get enough vitamins and minerals by just eating these most of the time?

A: That depends: How's your terpenoid intake lately? Are you getting enough polyphenols? What about anthocyanins and limonoids?

Vitamins and minerals get all the attention, but phytonutrients—the tens of thousands of plant-based micronutrients found in our food—are just as important. Some are anti-inflammatory, others help us battle microbes, and still more play a role in cancer prevention or help protect us from diabetes and heart disease.

And each individual plant has its own unique profile of phyto-nutrients. When we limit ourselves to a handful of regulars (even if those regulars are superstars like oranges or carrots), we're not getting the full range of nutrients that empower our bodies. On your next shopping trip, pick up even one fruit or vegetable you wouldn't normally eat. If you haven't enjoyed sunchokes, sorrel, rapini, chard, or black-eyed peas, give them a try. Or pick up an exotic, imported fruit like guava, cherimoya, horned melon, or kumquat. Rank them 1–5 on flavor and see if you don't find a new favorite to alternate with that Granny Smith apple.

Q: I sit all day at work, and I know that's not good for me. But I go to the gym several times a week and try to walk a lot as well. Am I in the clear?

A: Yes, as long as you're getting up from your chair every hour or so. A combination of regular exercise (especially if you follow the

Whole Body Fitness Plan) and just plain walking around is enough to keep the big muscles of your legs working. And here's a cool fact you probably didn't know: Every time you get up from your desk and your muscles contract, they secrete peptides called myokines, which enter the bloodstream and help protect against inflammation. The more time you spend on your feet, the more myokines your muscles release, and the more helpful they can be in fighting disease.

So on top of your fitness routine, don't let more than an hour or so go by without getting up out of your seat—no matter how intense your workday:

- Take your calls standing up. Not only does it get you up and moving, but standing for calls is an old trick businesspeople use to make themselves sound stronger, bolder, more energetic. That's you!

- Use a stand-up desk whenever possible. Hemingway wrote his greatest masterpieces standing up. You can gain mastery over your inbox from the same position.

- In the office? Walk to a colleague's desk instead of calling or emailing.

- On a long call? Put the phone on speaker or use a headset and get up and move a bit.

- Stretch and strengthen periodically. Keep a resistance band nearby and put it to use: Stand with both feet on the middle of the band and hold one end of the band in each hand. Then bend your elbows and curl your hands up to your shoulders. The wider your stance, the more resistance you'll get.

Chapter 14

Whole Body Recipes

Super Delicious Meals and
Snacks for the Whole Family

There are plenty of ways to supercharge your nutrition, reduce empty calories, and eat an overall healthier diet. But the easiest, most proven way of all comes down to three simple words: Cook at home.

As you've read repeatedly throughout this book, loading your diet with nutritionally dense food is more important than cutting calories. So it makes sense that you—and not some anonymous line cook at your local chain restaurant—should be the one in charge of what goes into your body.

When we eat at restaurants, our plates tend to be stacked much higher with saturated fat and sodium. In fact, preparing a meal at home is an automatic junk-caloric reduction: We consume an average of 200 calories more when we go out to eat than we do when we prepare all our meals at home, according to a University of Illinois study. And you already know that 200 fewer calories a day is our target to stop age-related waistline creep. Another study found that we eat fewer empty calories when we cook at home, regardless of whether or not we are consciously trying to manage our weight.

In this chapter, we present an array of recipes that are designed to meet the nutritional guidelines of the Whole Body Reset. That means they're packed with protein and fiber as well as vitamins, minerals, and phytochemicals, and have minimal unnecessary, empty calories so you can fulfill your body's nutritional needs without thinking. You'll find recipes for cooked and no-cook breakfasts; smoothies and protein shakes; lunch and dinner entrees; sides, salads, and soups; sauces and dressings (for those who want to take their cooking and taste buds to the next level); and yummy, nutrition-packed snacks.

Most of these recipes can easily be converted into vegetarian versions, simply by substituting meat with tofu, tempeh, or other plant-based proteins. You can also make easy substitutions if you're gluten or dairy free. As you'll see, many of the recipes are already naturally vegetarian, vegan, gluten free, or dairy free. But if you are avoiding animal products, or even just dairy products, it's important to make sure you're getting enough protein—particularly the amino acid leucine. Soy-based foods like tofu are among the top vegetable sources of leucine, as are kidney beans, watercress, spinach, and turnip greens. Spirulina, a form of algae you can find in health food stores, is particularly rich in this essential amino acid. Of course, you could easily follow this program without bothering with a single one of these recipes. Indeed, as you read in Chapter 9, you could probably eat fast food every single day and still manage to hit your nutritional marks. But isn't it great to know that whenever you're stumped for what to eat, the perfect meal or snack is yours to make?

A few quick notes on nutritional impact:

❑ While each of these recipes has been reviewed using established nutritional analysis software (ESHA.com), the exact nutrient counts can vary depending on your preparation method, the exact product and brand used, and serving size.

❑ When there is more than one option for an ingredient—for example "sliced almonds or pine nuts," or "chicken or vegetable broth"—the nutritional data are based on the first item.

❑ One scoop of protein powder provides about 20 grams of protein. Recipes assume animal-based powder; using plant-based may alter the leucine and B12 content.

Breakfast

It's the most important meal of the day, and also the one that most of us fail to get right. Too many of us start the day with a doughnut and coffee or, if you're fancy, a croissant and cappuccino. Delicious, yes. Convenient, for sure. But low on muscle-preserving, fat-fighting protein and disease-fighting, hunger-taming fiber. And even those of us who believe we're doing the right thing by sprinkling blueberries on our oatmeal simply aren't getting enough muscle-preserving protein, no matter how healthy that breakfast seems. Remember: If you don't eat enough protein in the morning, you're probably going to be in muscle breakdown all day long.

Each of the breakfasts in this chapter will give you at least 25 to 30 grams of protein and 5 grams of fiber. And while calorie counting isn't a main thrust of this program, it makes sense to watch your portion size. Women should be eating about 350 to 450 calories at breakfast, and men about 500 to 550, but keep in mind these are rough estimates. You can adjust these recipes as needed to tweak the calories and protein up or down as you see fit.

Since mornings can be more than a little stressful, we're starting with a collection of toss-'em-together, no-cook breakfasts you can whip up in just minutes.

No-Cook Breakfasts

I know, I know, I can already hear you whine, "I don't have time for breakfast." These recipes reduce cooking time to zero. Your excuses are now null and void.

The Waffle Cottage
(Vegetarian)

If you thought waffles were off the menu, you were wrong! A frozen waffle is the equivalent of eating a slice of bread; as long as you're starting with a whole grain waffle, you're in a good place.

1 SERVING

1 whole grain toaster waffle
¾ cup 1% cottage cheese
1 cup raspberries

10 whole almonds
1 teaspoon hemp seeds
1 teaspoon ground flax seeds

1. Toast the waffle as indicated on package.

2. Layer the cottage cheese, berries, nuts, and seeds on top.

NUTRITIONAL IMPACT: 29 g protein, 14 g fat, 36 g carbohydrates, 10 g fiber, 307 mg calcium, 484 mg potassium, 880 mg sodium, 1.37 mcg B12, 2.12 g leucine, 32 mg vitamin C, 372 calories

Wasa'p, New York?

A traditional Sunday-morning bagel with smoked salmon is common in New York City, but it's woefully low in fiber. Here's how to get your brunch on and still get the fiber you need: Serve this with a cup of melon (or fruit of your choice) and the *New York Times*. (Some people like to add capers, which are delicious but add a lot more sodium to an already high-sodium dish.)

1 SERVING

2 tablespoons cream cheese
2 Wasa crackers
2 slices tomato

4 ounces smoked salmon
1 cup cubes or 1 slice of melon

1. Spread a thin layer of cream cheese on both crackers.

2. Top the crackers with slices of tomatoes and salmon.

3. Serve with melon on the side.

NUTRITIONAL IMPACT (includes melon): 27 g protein, 15 g fat, 49 g carbohydrates, 10 g fiber, 69 mg calcium, 884 mg potassium, 1,097 mg sodium, 3.76 mcg B12, 0.21 g leucine, 35 mg vitamin C, 427 calories

Fun Fact

NOW LOOK HERE: Melon is a top source of two phytonutrients that support eye health: lutein and zeaxanthin.

Oatmeal

Oatmeal is a traditional healthy breakfast, but the vast majority of those who enjoy an oatmeal breakfast won't reach their morning protein goals. To help you make the most of your morning oats, we've specified toppings, amounts, and cooking directions (such as cooking the oats in milk instead of water) to be sure you get the protein you need.

These three approaches to oatmeal give you different ways to achieve the protein and fiber targets you should be looking for at every breakfast.

Many oats are gluten free; look for "gluten-free" on the packaging.

Muscled-Up Oats with Blueberries, Almonds, and Hemp Seeds

(Gluten-free, vegetarian)

This recipe uses water to cook the oats in the traditional manner but boosts the protein content with a small amount of protein powder and hemp seeds.

1 SERVING

½ cup water
½ cup rolled oats
½ scoop protein powder

1 cup blueberries
2 tablespoons sliced almonds
3 tablespoons hemp seeds

1. In a small pot, bring the water to a boil over medium heat. Add the oats.

2. Stir constantly until the oats have absorbed most of the water, about 5 minutes.

3. Mix in the protein powder.

4. Top with the blueberries, almonds, and hemp seeds.

NUTRITIONAL IMPACT: 31 g protein, 23 g fat, 54 g carbohydrates, 11 g fiber, 134 mg calcium, 422 mg potassium, 28 mg sodium, 0.38 mcg B12, 0.22 g leucine, 14 mg vitamin C, 529 calories

Fun Fact

A GARDEN WEASEL FOR YOUR ARTERIES: Beta-glucan is the soluble fiber in oats that reduces LDL (the "bad") and total cholesterol levels, especially in people with diabetes.

Milky Oats with Strawberries, Hemp Seeds, and Peanut Butter

(Gluten-free, vegetarian)

If you don't want to mess with protein powders, another easy way to add protein to oatmeal is to cook the oats in milk. And we can't say enough about the nutritional power of hemp seeds, which provide not only a remarkable amount of protein (more than 3 grams per tablespoon) but monounsaturated fatty acids as well.

1 SERVING

1 cup 1% milk
½ cup oats
½ cup strawberries, sliced

2 tablespoons hemp seeds
1 tablespoon plus 1 teaspoon peanut butter

1. In a medium pot, bring the milk to almost boiling over medium-high heat. Add the oats.

2. Stir constantly until the oatmeal has absorbed most of the milk, about 5 minutes.

3. Add the strawberries, hemp seeds, and peanut butter, and mix all ingredients together well.

NUTRITIONAL IMPACT: 25 g protein, 26 g fat, 51 g carbohydrates, 7 g fiber, 348 mg calcium, 742 mg potassium, 201 mg sodium, 1.15 mcg B12, 1.07 g leucine, 42 mg vitamin C, 520 calories

Oats While You Sleep
(Gluten-free, vegetarian)

Rushed in the morning? Use a jar to prepare these overnight oats that are ready to go the next day. The milk that saturates your oats overnight will give you the protein boost you need. You can substitute a plant-based "milk" like soy or pea milk—just make sure it has protein (so do not use almond or rice milk).

1 SERVING

1 cup 1% milk
½ cup rolled oats
¼ cup fresh blackberries

2 tablespoons hemp seeds
1 tablespoon chunky peanut butter

1. Place all ingredients in a bowl or jar and mix together.

2. Allow to sit overnight in the refrigerator. You can eat cold or microwave for 30 to 60 seconds if you prefer hot.

NUTRITIONAL IMPACT: 25 g protein, 23 g fat, 51 g carbohydrates, 8 g fiber, 346 mg calcium, 708 mg potassium, 188 mg sodium, 1.15 mcg B12, 0.97 g leucine, 8 mg vitamin C, 498 calories

Tips and Secrets

Less liquid makes for a thicker porridge but also reduces the protein. Add more liquid if you prefer. Experiment with different toppings and mix-ins.

Smoothies and Protein Drinks

A blender can do more than just punch your ticket to Margaritaville. It's also a powerful tool for boosting nutrition, giving you a delicious, dessert-like drink in about sixty seconds. While smoothies make breakfast fast and easy, they can also provide a terrific meal substitute at any time of the day. Use Greek yogurt or whey protein powder for a fast infusion of muscle-preserving nutrition. If you're looking for a vegan option, you can use vegan protein powder and a milk alternative; we recommend soy milk, which is higher in leucine content than other dairy substitutes, or pea protein, which also comes with a complete array of amino acids and has been shown in studies to be just as effective in muscle-building as whey protein.[1] (See page 127 for a full table with dairy milk alternatives.)

For each recipe, start by adding the liquid ingredients first, to make blending easier. Blend ingredients together for about a minute, until smooth. Add water or ice, or use frozen fruit, to change consistency or temperature (ice and frozen fruit create a thicker smoothie). If you're freezing bananas, remove the peels first; otherwise they will freeze into little impenetrable Kevlar vests. You can slice fruit before it's frozen; if slicing after, first run your knife under hot water.

Kale and Hearty Smoothie
(Gluten-free, vegetarian)

Although this smoothie recipe recommends adding the oats to create a full meal in a glass, you could cook the oats to eat separately and drink the smoothie without them, or skip the oats and have a slice of toast with avocado with your smoothie instead.

1 SERVING

1 cup 1% milk
½ cup plain low-fat Greek
  yogurt
1 cup frozen strawberries, sliced

½ small banana, sliced
⅓ cup oats
½ cup fresh kale, chopped

Place all the ingredients in a blender and blend until smooth.

NUTRITIONAL IMPACT: 25 g protein, 7 g fat, 56 g carbohydrates, 7 g fiber, 487 mg calcium, 1,028 mg potassium, 152 mg sodium, 1.74 mcg B12, 1.4 g leucine, 99 mg vitamin C, 374 calories

Super Immunity Smoothie
(Gluten-free, vegetarian)

During the onset of COVID-19, AARP spoke with experts on immunity to find the perfect smoothie to help regulate a healthy immune system. Turns out any recipe that includes probiotics (from kefir or yogurt), as well as plenty of fiber and phytonutrients (from berries, seeds, greens, and/or nut butters), will help support the immune system. This smoothie has an added protein boost from the protein powder.

1 SERVING

1 cup plain vitamin D–fortified kefir

½ medium fresh or frozen banana (for sweetness and creaminess)

1 cup frozen strawberries (or use mango or pineapple instead, or in combination)

1 tablespoon almond butter

1 cup fresh spinach leaves

1 teaspoon chia seeds

1 scoop whey isolate protein powder (you can use plant-based instead)

Place all the ingredients in a blender and blend until smooth.

NUTRITIONAL IMPACT: 40 g protein, 13 g fat, 43 g carbohydrates, 7 g fiber, 593 mg calcium, 1,249 mg potassium, 216 mg sodium, 1.54 mcg B12, 0.26 g leucine, 51 mg vitamin C, 444 calories

Fun Fact

CHA-CHA-CHA-CHIA! Chia seeds provide protein, omega-3 fatty acids, and fiber along with calcium, iron, and phytonutrients. And yes, they were the same used for those chia pets popular in the 1990s!

The Greek Banana Smoothie
(Gluten-free, vegetarian)

This smoothie is actually higher in carbohydrates than most of the other recipes due to the addition of applesauce. It's perfect to consume after a strenuous morning workout.

1 SERVING

½ cup water
½ cup applesauce
⅔ cup plain low-fat Greek yogurt
1 small banana
¼ cup rolled oats

½ teaspoon vanilla extract
¼ teaspoon ground cinnamon
1 cup fresh kale
1 tablespoon ground flax seeds
1 tablespoon hemp seeds

Place all the ingredients in a blender and blend until smooth.

NUTRITIONAL IMPACT: 25 g protein, 13 g fat, 65 g carbohydrates, 10 g fiber, 405 mg calcium, 634 mg potassium, 104 mg sodium, 0 mcg B12, 0.34 g leucine, 36 mg vitamin C, 466 calories

Fun Fact

HIT THE GROUND: Flax seeds are high in omega-3 fatty acids, fiber, and protein. But they're hard to digest, so opt for ground flax seeds to maximize your benefits.

"Dessert for Breakfast" Smoothie
(Gluten-free, vegetarian)

So delicious you may want to serve it in smaller portions as a dessert, but trust us, it's really a delivery system for powerful health-boosting nutrients.

1 SERVING

½ cup 1% milk

½ cup plain low-fat Greek yogurt

1 tablespoon unsweetened cocoa powder

1½ tablespoons peanut butter

1 small fresh or frozen banana

1 tablespoon avocado

2 teaspoons hemp seeds

Handful of ice (more based on preference)

Dash of ground cinnamon

Place all the ingredients in a blender and blend until smooth.

NUTRITIONAL IMPACT: 25 g protein, 22 g fat, 44 g carbohydrates, 7 g fiber, 308 mg calcium, 989 mg potassium, 198 mg sodium, 1.16 mcg B12, 1.12 g leucine, 11 mg vitamin C, 440 calories

Orange Crush Smoothie

(Gluten-free, vegetarian)

Super refreshing for warm summer mornings or whenever you want a light citrus boost.

1 SERVING

½ cup water
3 tablespoons orange juice
1 cup plain low-fat Greek
    yogurt
½ cup frozen peaches

½ banana (fresh or frozen)
2 tablespoons ground flax seeds
1 scoop vanilla protein powder
Handful of ice

Place all the ingredients in a blender and blend until smooth.

NUTRITIONAL IMPACT: 36 g protein, 13 g fat, 45 g carbohydrates, 8 g fiber, 325 mg calcium, 918 mg potassium, 177 mg sodium, 1.18 mcg B12, 1.4 g leucine, 114 mg vitamin C, 422 calories

Green Like Money Smoothie
(Gluten-free, vegetarian)

It's just as healthy as it looks; spinach gives this morning protein punch a green-juice vibe, but don't worry, it's still delicious.

1 SERVING

½ cup water
2 tablespoons orange juice
½ cup plain low-fat Greek yogurt
1 cup frozen spinach

⅓ cup blueberries (fresh or frozen)
¼ cup fresh kiwi (about 1 kiwi)
2 tablespoons ground flax seeds
1 scoop vanilla protein powder

Place all the ingredients in a blender and blend until smooth.

NUTRITIONAL IMPACT: 33 g protein, 11 g fat, 42 g carbohydrates, 14 g fiber, 511 mg calcium, 692 mg potassium, 337 mg sodium, 0.59 mcg B12, 0.78 g leucine, 77 mg vitamin C, 377 calories

SOLID PERFORMER: Spinach is high in nitrates, which help muscles relax and improve blood flow.

Pom-Pom Smoothie

(Gluten-free, vegetarian)

Go immune system, go! The mixed berries and pomegranate juice make this drink especially high in immune-supporting vitamin C.

1 SERVING

1 cup frozen mixed berries
½ cup plain low-fat Greek yogurt
¼ cup pomegranate juice

1 scoop vanilla protein powder
2 tablespoons hemp seeds
⅓ cup ice

Place all the ingredients in a blender and blend until smooth.

NUTRITIONAL IMPACT: 28 g protein, 14 g fat, 35 g carbohydrates, 7 g fiber, 170 mg calcium, 484 mg potassium, 134 mg sodium, 0.59 mcg B12, 0.6 g leucine, 10 mg vitamin C, 367 calories

Fun Fact

"HIGH" IMPACT: Hemp seeds pack a high protein punch for such a small package: 2 tablespoons provide 6 grams of protein. (And no, despite coming from the same species of plant as marijuana, hemp seeds can't get you high.)

The Right Side of the Bed Smoothie

(Gluten-free, vegetarian)

The green leaves of spinach and kale boost the folate content in this morning drink, giving your morning mood a boost. Studies show higher levels of this vitamin are consistent with lower levels of depression.[2] Healthy body, healthy brain!

1 SERVING

¾ cup plain low-fat Greek yogurt
¼ cup (2 ounces) fresh spinach
¼ cup (2 ounces) fresh kale
½ cup pineapple
½ medium banana
Dash of honey (¼ teaspoon)
1 scoop vanilla protein powder
⅓ cup ice

Place all the ingredients in a blender and blend until smooth.

NUTRITIONAL IMPACT: 30 g protein, 6 g fat, 45 g carbohydrates, 6 g fiber, 359 mg calcium, 1,035 mg potassium, 224 mg sodium, 0.88 mcg B12, 0.96 g leucine, 130 mg vitamin C, 340 calories

Creamy Dreamy Smoothie Bowl
(Gluten-free, dairy-free, vegetarian, vegan)

Tofu not only adds protein (10 grams in ½ cup!), but also creates a very creamy texture, much like a milkshake. Frozen banana adds to the ice cream–like consistency; freeze it when bright yellow, perhaps with some brown spots, to add sweetness.

If you want to drink this smoothie, rather than spoon it, increase the amount of plant-based milk to ¾ to 1 cup. If you prefer, the hemp seeds and berries can be blended in rather than used as toppings.

1 SERVING

Base:

½ cup unsweetened vanilla almond milk or other plant-based milk

½ cup (4 ounces) tofu

1 tablespoon almond butter

1 frozen banana, sliced

1 tablespoon unsweetened cocoa powder (optional)

Toppings:

3 tablespoons hemp seeds

½ cup (total amount) frozen raspberries and blueberries, thawed or microwaved so that the berries exude their juices

1. For the base: In a blender, blend all the ingredients in the order listed. Start the blender on low, and gradually increase speed until everything is combined and consistency is smooth. You might need to stop the blender occasionally to scrape down the sides and bottom with a rubber spatula. If things are not moving along, add splashes of milk to the blender to get everything going.

2. Pour the base into a bowl and top with hemp seeds and berries.

NUTRITIONAL IMPACT: 26 g protein, 31 g fat, 42 g carbohydrates, 11 g fiber, 465 mg calcium, 876 mg potassium, 136 mg sodium, 0 mcg B12, 0.37 g leucine, 19 mg vitamin C, 507 calories

Cooked Breakfasts

On days when you're feeling ambitious, or on weekends when the house is hungry and looking to you for sustenance, these recipes will satisfy both your nutritional needs and your gourmet instincts.

Scramblin' Around Tofu

(Gluten-free, dairy-free, vegetarian, vegan)

Here's a clever way to introduce tofu to skeptics who think this creamy block of vegan nutrition is a Commie plot to undermine American masculinity. In fact, tofu is an effective protein delivery system, and this recipe will jump-start your muscle-building morning.

1 SERVING

1 tablespoon extra-virgin olive oil
½ cup mushrooms, chopped
1 cup kale, chopped
½ red bell pepper, diced
¼ cup onion, diced
½ cup soft tofu, drained and crumbled

½ teaspoon garlic powder (or fresh minced garlic)
2 tablespoons nutritional yeast
Salt and pepper to taste
2 slices whole wheat toast (with toast this recipe is not gluten-free)

1. In a medium sauté pan, heat the olive oil over medium heat.

2. Add the mushrooms, kale, bell peppers, and onion and sauté 5 to 7 minutes, until onions are translucent.

3. Add the tofu, garlic, yeast, salt, and pepper, and sauté for 3 to 5 minutes.

4. Serve the tofu mixture over or alongside 2 slices of toast or grain of your choice—cooked oats, leftover brown rice or quinoa, or even baked new potatoes.

NUTRITIONAL IMPACT (includes 2 slices of whole wheat toast): 30 g protein, 21 g fat, 50 g carbohydrates, 15 g fiber, 685 mg calcium, 878 mg potassium, 370 mg sodium, 24 mcg B12, 0.11 g leucine, 118 mg vitamin C, 494 calories

Fun Fact

IN LIVING COLOR: Red and green bell peppers are the same plant. But red peppers are sweeter—and have twice as much vitamin C—because they're allowed to ripen on the vine.

Protein-Punch Pancakes

(Gluten-free, vegetarian)

Pancakes are usually just an excuse to eat cake for breakfast—there's little difference between the two. But these stovetop diskettes are veritable flying Frisbees of fitness. Flannel shirt and lumberjack axe optional.

1 SERVING (5 THIN PANCAKES, ABOUT 3 INCHES IN DIAMETER)

1 egg
1 egg white
½ cup plain nonfat Greek yogurt
½ cup rolled oats
½ teaspoon baking powder

½ medium banana
½ teaspoon vanilla extract
½ cup frozen blueberries
Olive oil cooking spray
Cinnamon to taste
Honey to taste (optional)

1. Place all ingredients up to the blueberries in a blender and blend until smooth.

2. Mix in the berries.

3. Coat a skillet with the cooking spray and place over medium heat.

4. Spoon the batter onto the hot skillet and cook until golden, then flip, cooking the other side until golden brown.

5. Sprinkle with cinnamon and, if desired, honey to taste. (Calories for honey are not included in nutritional analysis.)

NUTRITIONAL IMPACT: 31 g protein, 8 g fat, 59 g carbohydrates, 8 g fiber, 486 mg calcium, 739 mg potassium, 208 mg sodium, 1.29 mcg B12, 1.1 g leucine, 7 mg vitamin C, 434 calories

Tips and Secrets

- Put the liquid ingredients in the blender first for easier blending, or you can simply mix everything in a bowl.

- Flip the pancakes when bubbles appear on the surface and the edges start to look dry. (But it never hurts to peek under to make sure!)

Más Macho Nacho Supreme

(Gluten-free, vegetarian)

A nontraditional breakfast and a twist on huevos rancheros, this can be a welcome change and fun for the whole family. The portion below is for one; just multiply based on your family size!

1 SERVING

10 tortilla chips
¼ cup part-skim mozzarella, shredded
¼ cup low-sodium black beans, drained and rinsed
½ red bell pepper, diced
Olive oil cooking spray

1 egg
1 egg white
¼ cup tomatoes, diced
¼ avocado, diced
1 tablespoon chopped cilantro (optional)

1. Preheat oven or toaster oven to 350°F.

2. Place the tortilla chips on a rimmed baking sheet; you can line it with aluminum foil.

3. Sprinkle the chips with cheese, beans, and red pepper.

4. Bake just a few minutes, until cheese melts.

5. While the chips bake, in a nonstick skillet or a skillet coated with cooking spray, scramble the eggs over medium heat.

6. Remove the chips from the oven and slide onto a plate. Top with the scrambled egg, tomato, avocado, and cilantro.

NUTRITIONAL IMPACT: 27 g protein, 24 g fat, 39 g carbohydrates, 10 g fiber, 266 mg calcium, 903 mg potassium, 500 mg sodium, 0.45 mcg B12, 1.45 g leucine, 107 mg vitamin C, 485 calories

The Bogart Bowl

(Gluten-free, vegetarian)

It's hard-boiled. Get it?

1 SERVING

Cooking oil spray
1 cup spinach
¼ cup chopped white onion
Salt and pepper to taste

⅓ cup brown basmati rice, cooked according to package directions
3 hard-boiled eggs, halved
¼ avocado, chopped

1. In a nonstick skillet or a skillet coated with cooking spray, sauté the spinach and onion over medium heat. Season with salt and pepper.

2. Place the rice in a bowl and top with the sautéed vegetables, hard-boiled eggs, and avocado.

NUTRITIONAL IMPACT: 25 g protein, 21 g fat, 55 g carbohydrates, 7 g fiber, 108 mg calcium, 624 mg potassium, 207 mg sodium, 1.47 mcg B12, 0.08 g leucine, 16 mg vitamin C, 483 calories

Fun Fact

HOT TEARS: It's the sulfuric acid in onions that makes you weep. To avoid the tears, try cutting the onion under running water or chilling the onion before cutting it.

Lunch and Dinner Entrees

We haven't discriminated between lunch and dinner options, because, as you've learned from previous chapters, you need to regularly infuse your body with high-nutrition, moderate-calorie meals throughout the day, rather than eating one big, protein-laden dinner as most Americans do. So lunch can and should be about the same size as dinner. (In fact, in an ideal world your lunch would actually be a tiny bit larger than your dinner, as we look to shift calories toward earlier in the day.)

Each of these recipes is a complete meal, meeting all your nutritional requirements—at least 25 to 30 grams of protein and 5 grams of fiber. In most cases, we've paired a protein dish with a side vegetable, giving your body everything it needs.

If some of these multistep recipes seem time-consuming or overwhelming, make as much as you can ahead of time.

Pumpkin It Up! Chili with Take It for Pomegranate Salad

A super meal for any day, not just Super Bowl Sunday. The addition of pumpkin provides velvety thickness and unique sweet/savoriness to the chili, resulting in an awesome dish without excess meat. To balance out this fiber-packed bowl of comfort, enjoy with a whole grain roll or a serving of whole grain crackers and Take It for Pomegranate Salad (or substitute any salad or leafy green of your choice).

Pumpkin It Up! Chili
(Gluten-free)

4 SERVINGS

1½ tablespoons avocado oil
(or peanut oil)
¼ pound ground turkey
(93% lean) or ground chicken
1 medium red onion, finely diced
1 small jalapeño pepper,
minced, with some seeds
2½ cups low-sodium chicken
broth
1 can (15 ounces) pure pumpkin
1 can (14½ ounces) no-salt-
added crushed fire-roasted
tomatoes

1½ tablespoons chili powder
¼ teaspoon ground cinnamon
½ teaspoon sea salt, or to taste
1 can (15 ounces) low-sodium
red kidney beans, drained
and rinsed
1 cup shredded Monterey Jack
cheese
½ cup fresh whole cilantro
leaves

1. Heat the avocado oil in a stockpot on medium-high heat. Add the turkey, onion, and jalapeño and sauté until the turkey is finely crumbled and onion is softened, about 4 minutes.

2. Stir in the broth, pumpkin, tomatoes (with liquid), chili powder, cinnamon, and salt and bring to a boil over high heat.

3. Reduce heat to medium and cook uncovered for 15 minutes.

4. Stir in the beans and cook until they're heated through and chili is desired consistency, about 5 minutes more. Adjust seasoning.

5. Ladle the chili into individual bowls, sprinkle with cheese and cilantro, and serve.

CHILI NUTRITIONAL IMPACT PER SERVING (using ground turkey; includes garnish): 25 g protein, 18 g fat, 39 g carbohydrates, 13 g fiber, 291 mg calcium, 1,201 mg potassium, 793 mg sodium, 0.38 mcg B12, 1.5 g leucine, 17 mg vitamin C, 392 calories

Take It for Pomegranate Salad

(Gluten-free, dairy-free, vegetarian)

4 SERVINGS

1½ tablespoons pomegranate juice (or other fruit juice)

1½ tablespoons apple cider vinegar

1 tablespoon extra-virgin olive oil

⅛ teaspoon sea salt

½ teaspoon ground black pepper

1 package (5 ounces) baby arugula or mixed salad greens

½ cup fresh pomegranate seeds or dried tart cherries

1. In a large bowl, whisk together the pomegranate juice, vinegar, avocado oil, salt, and pepper. Add the arugula and toss.

2. Sprinkle with the pomegranate seeds to serve.

SALAD NUTRITIONAL IMPACT PER SERVING: 1 g protein, 4 g fat, 18 g carbohydrates, 1 g fiber, 26 mg calcium, 190 mg potassium, 87 mg sodium, 0 mcg B12, 0 g leucine, 8 mg vitamin C, 106 calories

TOTAL NUTRITIONAL IMPACT PER SERVING: 26 g protein, 22 g fat, 57 g carbohydrates, 14 g fiber, 317 mg calcium, 1,391 mg potassium, 880 mg sodium, 0.38 mcg B12, 1.5 g leucine, 25 mg vitamin C, 498 calories

RECIPE VARIATIONS

In place of the ground turkey or chicken, low-sodium chicken broth, and garnish of shredded Monterey Jack cheese and cilantro leaves, try these variations:

- Grass-fed ground beef sirloin, low-sodium beef broth, and garnish of cheddar cheese and parsley leaves
- 1 cup finely chopped Baby Bella mushrooms, low-sodium vegetable broth, and garnish of plant-based cheese and sliced scallions

GOT LEFTOVERS?

Make Cincinnati-style chili by serving warmed chili over whole wheat spaghetti. Or ladle the chili over a baked potato.

Tips and Secrets

Make your own chili seasoning in advance by mixing together the chili powder, cinnamon, and salt. Preparing the vinaigrette in advance is also a time-saver.

Open Sesame Chicken and Veggies Stir-Fry with Citrus Brown Rice

What's better than Chinese takeout? This is! And it's so easy—you just roast everything on sheet pans—no wok necessary! The chicken is deliciously moist since the recipe calls for chicken thighs. You can vary the veggies to make it your own. Pair it with Citrus Brown Rice or any steamed whole grain of choice—even ninety-second microwave brown rice is A-OK. If you go with a plain grain, just stir in some orange zest to keep the distinctive and aromatic citrusy flair.

Open Sesame Chicken and Veggies Stir-Fry

(Gluten-free, dairy-free)

4 SERVINGS

3 tablespoons reduced-sodium tamari (soy sauce); if you're gluten free, be sure to use gluten-free tamari

2 tablespoons sesame oil

2 tablespoons natural creamy almond butter or peanut butter

1 tablespoon rice vinegar or cider vinegar

1 tablespoon freshly grated ginger

2 large cloves garlic, minced

¼ cup orange juice

1 pound boneless, skinless chicken thighs, cut into 1-inch cubes

5 cups (packed) sliced fresh bok choy

2 large red bell peppers, sliced

1 small hot chile pepper, minced, with some seeds

(RECIPE CONTINUES ON NEXT PAGE)

Garnish:

2 tablespoons roasted or toasted sesame seeds

½ cup fresh whole cilantro leaves or sliced scallions

1. Preheat oven to 450°F.

2. In a large mixing bowl, whisk together the tamari, sesame oil, almond butter, vinegar, ginger, and garlic until combined. Whisk in the orange juice.

3. Add the chicken and gently toss with tongs to coat. Add the bok choy, bell peppers, and chile pepper and toss to coat.

4. Transfer the mixture evenly onto two large rimmed baking sheets and spread out into single layers. Roast until the chicken is well done and vegetables begin to brown, about 25 minutes.

5. Sprinkle with sesame seeds and cilantro. Serve with additional tamari, if desired.

STIR-FRY NUTRITIONAL IMPACT PER SERVING (includes garnish): 29 g protein, 18 g fat, 14 g carbohydrates, 4 g fiber, 138 mg calcium, 561 mg potassium, 706 mg sodium, 0 mcg B12, 0.22 g leucine, 175 mg vitamin C, 326 calories

Tips and Secrets

For the stir-fry, make the sauce in advance by combining the tamari, sesame oil, almond butter, vinegar, ginger, garlic, and orange juice in a jar; cover, shake, and store in the fridge for up to a week. Cut up veggies in advance, too—or just pick up pre-prepped vegetables from your local market.

Citrus Brown Rice

(Gluten-free, dairy-free, vegetarian, vegan)

4 SERVINGS

1 cup dry brown basmati rice
1⅓ cups low-sodium vege-
    table broth (or water; for a
    non-vegetarian version, use
    chicken broth)
½ cup orange juice

⅛ teaspoon sea salt, or to taste
2 teaspoons orange zest
    (1 medium orange provides
    about ¼ cup juice and
    3 teaspoons orange zest)

1. In a small saucepan, combine all the ingredients and bring to a boil over high heat.

2. Cover, reduce heat to low, and simmer until the rice is just cooked through, about 40 minutes.

3. Remove from the heat and let stand, covered, for 10 minutes to complete the cooking process.

RICE NUTRITIONAL IMPACT PER SERVING: 5 g protein, 2 g fat, 38 g carbohydrates, 3 g fiber, 5 mg calcium, 64 mg potassium, 121 mg sodium, 0 mcg B12, 0 g leucine, 17 mg vitamin C, 172 calories

TOTAL NUTRITIONAL IMPACT PER SERVING: 34 g protein, 20 g total fat, 52 g carbohydrates, 7 g fiber, 143 mg calcium, 625 mg potassium, 827 mg sodium, 0 mcg B12, 0.22 g leucine, 192 mg vitamin C, 498 calories

RECIPE VARIATIONS

In place of the chicken cubes, sliced bok choy, and sesame seeds, try these variations:

- Extra-firm tofu or tempeh, broccoli florets, and roasted, chopped peanuts
- Precooked shrimp (stir in 5 minutes before end of roasting), cut asparagus or green beans, and toasted sliced almonds

GOT LEFTOVERS?

Mix the stir-fry with the rice and simply reheat. Or you can crisp it up in a skillet or wok with a drizzling of oil to make fried rice.

Fun Fact

HAVE A RICE DAY! Brown basmati rice, originally grown in India and Pakistan, is a long-grained variety that has a distinct nutty flavor and delivers fiber, which helps you feel full and satisfied, plus vitamin E, magnesium, copper, and folate.

Muscled-Up Pesto Pasta with Basil Turkey Meatballs

This plant-forward primavera is based on "pulse pasta"—pasta made from protein-rich sources such as chickpea or red lentil—and lightly dressed with pesto. So, it's an ultra-satisfying trio of plant protein, fiber, and healthy fats. (Try some different types of pulse pastas to find the one you like best; personally, I think chickpea tastes closest to regular wheat pasta.) You can make it with any seasonal non-starchy vegetables you like. To complete your meal, pair it with Basil Turkey Meatballs plus a side of fruit. The meatballs can be served as an appetizer, as a side dish, or on top of your bowl of primavera.

Muscled-Up Pesto Pasta
(Gluten-free, vegetarian)

4 SERVINGS

Pesto:

1½ cups packed fresh basil leaves

¼ cup chopped walnuts, preferably pan-toasted

2 tablespoons extra-virgin olive oil

2 large cloves garlic, chopped

1½ tablespoons lemon juice

⅛ teaspoon crushed red pepper flakes

½ teaspoon sea salt

2 tablespoons grated Parmesan cheese

Pasta:

8 ounces dry pulse pasta, such as red lentil or chickpea

1 tablespoon avocado oil or high-oleic sunflower oil

4 cups packed non-starchy vegetables, such as a mixture of broccoli florets, grape tomatoes, and sliced summer squash

¼ teaspoon sea salt

1. For the pesto: In a food processor, combine all the ingredients except the Parmesan cheese and pulse until finely chopped. Add the Parmesan cheese and puree until desired consistency. Set aside.

(RECIPE CONTINUES ON NEXT PAGE)

2. In a large saucepan, bring salted water three-quarters filled to a boil over high heat. Stir in the pasta and cook according to package directions (8 to 10 minutes; cooking times vary).

3. Meanwhile, in a large, deep cast-iron skillet or other nonstick skillet, heat the avocado oil over medium-high heat. Add the vegetables and salt and sauté until the vegetables are crisp-tender and browned, about 6 minutes.

4. Drain the pasta, quickly rinse under cold water for a few seconds just to stop the cooking process, and drain again. Then, in the dry saucepan or a large mixing bowl, toss the pasta with the pesto. Adjust seasoning to taste.

5. Transfer the pasta to a serving bowl or individual bowls, top with the sautéed vegetables, and serve.

PASTA NUTRITIONAL IMPACT PER SERVING: 15 g protein, 17 g fat, 40 g carbohydrates, 5 g fiber, 75 mg calcium, 622 mg potassium, 502 mg sodium, 0.04 mcg B12, 0.17 g leucine, 29 mg vitamin C, 362 calories

Basil Turkey Meatballs

4 SERVINGS

¼ cup fresh basil, chopped
¼ cup dry whole wheat bread crumbs
¼ cup Parmesan cheese, grated
¼ cup red onion, coarsely grated
1 large egg
2 cloves garlic, minced

2 teaspoons extra-virgin olive oil
¼ teaspoon plus ⅛ teaspoon sea salt
⅛ teaspoon crushed red pepper flakes, or to taste
6 ounces ground turkey (93% lean)

1. Preheat oven to 450°F and line a rimmed baking sheet with unbleached parchment paper.

2. In a medium bowl, stir together all the ingredients except the turkey until well combined. Add the turkey and combine until evenly combined.

3. Form the mixture into 12 meatballs, about 2 tablespoons each. Place onto the baking sheet.

4. Roast until well done, about 15 minutes, flipping over meatballs halfway through the roasting process. Serve.

MEATBALLS NUTRITIONAL IMPACT PER SERVING: 13 g protein, 8 g fat, 8 g carbohydrates, 1 g fiber, 60 mg calcium, 178 mg potassium, 359 mg sodium, 0.18 mcg B12, 0.27 g leucine, 2 mg vitamin C, 150 calories

TOTAL NUTRITIONAL IMPACT PER SERVING: 28 g protein, 25 g fat, 48 g carbohydrates, 6 g fiber, 135 mg calcium, 800 mg potassium, 861 mg sodium, 0.22 mcg B12, 0.44 g leucine, 31 mg vitamin C, 512 calories

RECIPE VARIATIONS

In place of the pulse pasta and walnuts, try these variations:

- Whole wheat pasta or gnocchi and pine nuts
- Zucchini noodles ("zoodles") and pistachios

GOT LEFTOVERS?

Enjoy as pasta salad. Squirt with lemon juice to liven it up. Sprinkle with chopped walnuts for bonus crunch.

Tips and Secrets

Pulse pasta can generally be found in the pasta aisle.

Make the pesto in advance, cover, and chill in the refrigerator for up to three days. Or use ⅔ cup of any pesto, including jarred basil pesto.

"I Ain't Cookin' Tonight" Taco Bowl with Pumpkin Seed Guac

This is a recipe for people who love to eat but hate to cook (or do dishes)! If you don't have leftover cooked veggies on hand, just dice two large, sweet bell peppers and enjoy them crisp and raw. And do eat the collard green leaves that form the "bowl"—they're not just décor. Serve this Tex-Mex creation at room temperature, rather than chilled, for the tastiest results. And pair it with Pumpkin Seed Guac—or simply add sliced avocado to each bowl. Roll up any remaining collard greens to dip in the guacamole.

"I Ain't Cookin' Tonight" Taco Bowl
(Gluten-free, vegetarian)

4 SERVINGS

8 large fresh collard greens or other large dark leafy greens such as Swiss chard or kale

1 can (15 ounces) black beans or pinto beans

2 cups frozen corn, thawed

1 pint grape tomatoes, halved

4 cups (packed) leftover roasted or grilled non-starchy vegetables, such as roasted cauliflower

½ small red onion, finely diced

1 cup finely diced cheddar cheese

½ cup fresh whole cilantro leaves

¾ teaspoon chipotle chili powder or taco seasoning

½ cup plain low-fat Greek yogurt

½ cup salsa verde

1. Wash the collard green leaves with cold water and pat dry. Cut off thick stems.

2. Line four dinner bowls with the collard greens.

3. Evenly divide and arrange all the ingredients in the leafy bowls except the salsa.

4. Serve the salsa on the side.

TACO BOWL NUTRITIONAL IMPACT PER SERVING: 22 g protein, 22 g fat, 63 g carbohydrates, 12 g fiber, 389 mg calcium, 369 mg potassium, 937 mg sodium, 0.51 mcg B12, 1.11 g leucine, 140 mg vitamin C, 509 calories

RECIPE VARIATIONS

You can replace the ¾ teaspoon chipotle chili powder with a mixture of ½ teaspoon smoked paprika + ⅛ teaspoon ground cayenne pepper + ⅛ teaspoon ground chili powder.

In place of the black or pinto beans, thawed frozen corn, and leftover roasted or grilled cooked vegetables like cauliflower, try these variations:

- Shredded rotisserie chicken breast meat, chilled brown rice or riced cauliflower, and roasted orange bell pepper
- Cubed leftover grilled grass-fed beef or pork, grilled corn cut off the cob, and grilled green bell peppers

Pumpkin Seed Guac

(Gluten-free, dairy-free, vegetarian, vegan)

4 SERVINGS

2 large avocados, peeled, pitted, and cubed

1½ tablespoons lime juice

¼ cup red onion, diced

¼ cup fresh cilantro, roughly chopped

½ small jalapeño pepper, minced, with seeds (optional)

½ teaspoon ground coriander

¼ teaspoon sea salt, or to taste

¼ cup shelled, roasted, and salted pumpkin seeds

1. In a medium bowl, gently stir together all the ingredients except the pumpkin seeds.

2. When ready to serve, stir the pumpkin seeds into the guacamole or sprinkle them on top.

GUAC NUTRITIONAL IMPACT PER SERVING: 5 g protein, 19 g fat, 11 g carbohydrates, 8 g fiber, 22 mg calcium, 518 mg potassium, 173 mg sodium, 0 mcg B12, 0.15 g leucine, 15 mg vitamin C, 210 calories

TOTAL NUTRITIONAL IMPACT PER SERVING: 27 g protein, 41 g fat, 74 g carbohydrates, 20 g fiber, 411 mg calcium, 887 mg potassium, 1,110 mg sodium, 0.51 mcg B12, 1.26 g leucine, 155 mg vitamin C, 719 calories

GOT LEFTOVERS?

Serve the guac with crudité for a snack, or use it as a spread on a sandwich, or on toast in the morning.

Tips and Secrets

Rather than attractively arranging all the ingredients in each leafy "bowl," cut up the greens into bite-sized pieces and stir everything together.

Fun Fact

MY SWEET GOURD: Just 1 ounce of protein-packed pumpkin seeds contains 37 percent of your recommended daily intake of muscle-building magnesium.

Scramblin' Around (with Fruit)
(Gluten-free, vegetarian)

This one-skillet meal is satisfying any time of day—just make sure you've got a skillet big enough to fit all of the ingredients! Enjoy this flavorful fix along with some in-season fresh fruit, perhaps a cup of berries.

4 SERVINGS

1 tablespoon plus 1½ teaspoons avocado oil or extra-virgin olive oil

1 large sweet potato with skin, cut into ½-inch cubes (about 3 cups)

4 scallions, thinly sliced, green and white parts separated

1 pint grape tomatoes

9 large eggs, lightly beaten

1 cup shredded Monterey Jack cheese

⅓ cup fresh cilantro, chopped

½ teaspoon sea salt, or to taste

1 package (5 ounces) baby spinach

24 corn tortilla chips

⅓ cup salsa or salsa verde

½ cup fresh strawberries

½ cup fresh blueberries

1. In a large, deep cast-iron skillet or other nonstick skillet (at least 12-inch diameter), heat 1 tablespoon of the oil over medium-high heat. Add the sweet potato and white parts of the scallions and sauté until the scallions are browned and the sweet potato is just cooked through, about 10 minutes. Add the tomatoes and sauté until warm, about 1 minute.

2. Reduce heat to low. Push the vegetables to the side of the skillet. Add the remaining oil to the center of the skillet. Then add the eggs, cheese, cilantro, green parts of the scallions, and salt and cook, gently folding the eggs until softly scrambled, about 2 minutes.

3. Remove from the heat and stir the spinach into the eggs and vegetables until just wilted, about 1 to 2 minutes more. Adjust seasoning, if desired.

(RECIPE CONTINUES ON NEXT PAGE)

4. To serve, stir in the tortilla chips or arrange on top. Drizzle with the salsa or serve it on the side.

5. Wash the strawberries and blueberries to accompany the dish.

NUTRITIONAL IMPACT PER SERVING (includes ½ cup fresh blueberries and ½ cup fresh strawberries): 25 g protein, 29 g fat, 32 g carbohydrates, 5 g fiber, 327 mg calcium, 440 mg potassium, 833 mg sodium, 1.24 mcg B12, 1.85 g leucine, 36 mg vitamin C, 477 calories

RECIPE VARIATIONS
In place of the sweet potato, grape tomatoes, and Monterey Jack cheese, try these variations:

- Red or blue potatoes, green bell pepper, and cheddar cheese
- Butternut squash, red bell pepper, and goat or cashew cheese

GOT LEFTOVERS?
Stuff some of the prepared scramble into a whole grain tortilla, roll up, and heat in the microwave to make an egg burrito.

Tips and Secrets

A day in advance, bake a sweet potato in the oven or microwave and chill; when ready to prepare the recipe, dice it up and sauté for about 3 minutes instead of 10.

Salmon Ahroooo-Gla!
with Rosemary Roasted
Butternut Squash

A salad worthy of the best steakhouse in town. If you want something fast for lunch, use a precooked piece of salmon, but for best effect, toss a nice piece of fresh fish on the grill. Make it a complete meal by using a slightly bigger piece of fish to up the protein quotient, or by pairing it with a side like Rosemary Roasted Butternut Squash. (Do make sure you plan ahead since the squash needs about 1½ hours in the oven.)

Salmon Ahroooo-Gla!

(Gluten-free)

4 SERVINGS

1 package (5 ounces) baby arugula

½ small red onion, thinly sliced

¼ cup white balsamic or champagne vinegar

3 tablespoons extra-virgin olive oil, divided

¼ teaspoon sea salt

1 teaspoon ground black pepper

10 ounces salmon filet, cut into 4 portions

2 large yellow bell peppers, cut into 4 or 5 large pieces each

¼ cup finely crumbled blue cheese

¼ cup sliced almonds or pine nuts, preferably pan-toasted

1. Heat a grill or grill pan over medium-high heat.

2. On a large platter or individual plates, arrange the arugula and onion; set aside.

3. In a liquid measuring cup or small bowl, whisk together the vinegar, 2 tablespoons of olive oil, salt, and pepper to make the vinaigrette; set aside.

4. Brush the salmon with the remaining 1 tablespoon of olive oil.

(RECIPE CONTINUES ON NEXT PAGE)

5. Grill the salmon (flesh side down first) and bell peppers, in batches if necessary, until the salmon is cooked through and peppers have rich char marks, about 4 to 5 minutes per side.

6. Thinly slice the bell peppers and arrange on the salad. Top with the salmon. Sprinkle everything with the vinaigrette, blue cheese, and nuts, and serve.

SALMON NUTRITIONAL IMPACT PER SERVING: 20 g protein, 26 g fat, 12 g carbohydrates, 2 g fiber, 147 mg calcium, 629 mg potassium, 374 mg sodium, 2.36 mcg B12, 1.43 g leucine, 176 mg vitamin C, 350 calories

Tips and Secrets

Make the vinaigrette in advance and store it in a jar in your fridge so it's ready whenever you are; it can be stored for weeks.

Wild or Not?

"Wild salmon" sounds awfully rugged and romantic, doesn't it? As though Ernest Hemingway himself somehow wrestled the silvery creature straight from the cold waters of Alaska and onto your plate? And it's definitely nutritionally superior— you get a much healthier balance of fats, and fewer overall calories, from wild-caught fish. That's one reason it costs more. But the nonprofit group Oceana collected samples of salmon from eighty-two restaurants and grocery stores and, after performing DNA testing, determined that much of it was mislabeled, with 69 percent of the errors consisting of farmed salmon being sold as more expensive wild salmon. Mislabeling tends to go up significantly in winter, when wild salmon is out of season.

RECIPE VARIATIONS

In place of the salmon filets, try these variations:

- Chicken filets or beefsteaks
- Large portobello mushroom caps (sprinkle with extra pine nuts)

GOT LEFTOVERS?

Any leftover salmon salad can be transformed into a tasty sandwich or wrap, even if the arugula is wilted.

Rosemary Roasted Butternut Squash

(Gluten-free, vegetarian)

4 SERVINGS

1 large (3 pounds) butternut squash, halved lengthwise and seeded (do not peel)

1½ teaspoons extra-virgin olive oil

2 teaspoons minced fresh rosemary or 1 teaspoon dried

1½ teaspoons sea salt

1½ teaspoons ground black pepper

1½ tablespoons crumbled blue cheese or pan-toasted pine nuts (or a mix, as counted in analysis)

1. Preheat oven to 375°F.

2. Brush the cut sides of the squash halves with the oil. Sprinkle with rosemary, salt, and pepper. Place on a large, rimmed baking sheet, cut sides facing up. Cover well with foil.

3. Roast for 45 minutes.

4. Remove the foil and roast until squash is fork tender and begins to brown, about 45 to 50 minutes more.

5. Sprinkle with the blue cheese (or pine nuts or mix, if using) and serve.

SQUASH NUTRITIONAL IMPACT PER SERVING: 5 g protein, 5 g fat, 41 g carbohydrates, 7 g fiber, 185 mg calcium, 1,218 mg potassium, 934 mg sodium, 0.04 mcg B12, 0.26 g leucine, 71 mg vitamin C, 200 calories

TOTAL NUTRITIONAL IMPACT PER SERVING: 550 calories, 25 g protein, 26 g fat, 53 g carbohydrates, 9 g fiber, 332 mg calcium, 1,847 mg potassium, 1,308 mg sodium, 2.4 mcg B12, 1.69 g leucine, 247 mg vitamin C

Lean Green Sardines
(Dairy-free)

This is classic Mediterranean-style eating. Salads that combine bread and tomatoes are called *panzanella*. If you don't like sardines, feel free to substitute another fish high in omega-3, such as salmon, trout, tuna, or mackerel. The salad also pairs nicely with grilled chicken or steak.

Some like the taste of raw kale, but others find it bitter. To tenderize raw kale, releasing the bitter taste, massage it with some of the dressing before adding the other ingredients. The massage, along with the acid from the vinegar and lemon juice, helps break down the fibers. (It might be fun to annoy waiters by asking them to massage your kale, but we are not responsible for any face-slapping that might ensue.)

4 SERVINGS

¾ cup sourdough bread, cut into cubes

2 cups spinach

2 cups kale, chopped

1 cup fresh red bell pepper, diced

1 cup cucumber, peeled, sliced, and cut into half moons

1½ cups cherry tomatoes

12 kalamata olives

¼ cup red onion, chopped

½ avocado, sliced

3 tablespoons chickpeas, drained and rinsed

¼ cup spearmint leaves

16 ounces sardines (fresh or canned)

Vinaigrette:

1 tablespoon balsamic vinegar

1 tablespoon lemon juice

1 clove garlic, finely chopped or grated (1 teaspoon)

¼ teaspoon dried oregano

2 tablespoons extra-virgin olive oil

¼ teaspoon crushed red pepper flakes

Salt and pepper to taste

(RECIPE CONTINUES ON NEXT PAGE)

1. Preheat oven to 350°F.

2. Bake the cubes of bread for 10 minutes. (You *do not* want cubes to get hard like croutons; they should resemble stale bread.)

3. While the bread is in the oven, make the vinaigrette. In a small bowl, combine all the ingredients and whisk well. For a creamier vinaigrette, use a blender. (This can also be done in a bowl using an immersion blender.)

4. In a large bowl, toss together all the salad ingredients except the sardines.

5. At least 10 minutes before serving (to allow bread time to absorb the vinaigrette), drizzle in the dressing and toss until all ingredients are well incorporated.

6. On a hot outdoor or indoor grill over medium heat, grill the sardines, about 2 minutes each side, looking for just a slight char and grill marks. Take the fish off the grill and cover with aluminum foil to keep warm. (Grilling is not necessary—you can use the sardines straight out of the can. But you'll find this extra step gives them a smoky crispiness that adds to the overall dish.)

7. Serve the salad topped with sardines, either family style or as individual portions.

NUTRITIONAL IMPACT PER SERVING: 36 g protein, 29 g fat, 37 g carbohydrates, 6 g fiber, 517 mg calcium, 1,061 mg potassium, 875 mg sodium, 10.14 mcg B12, 2.43 g leucine, 75 mg vitamin C, 549 calories

Tips and Secrets

Prepare the bread cubes the day before or use day-old (stale) bread.

Salmon-I-Am Salad

(Dairy-free)

Most of us consume barley only if we're drinking beer, but the high-fiber grain helps transform this protein-packed salad into a fast and satisfying meal.

4 SERVINGS

1 cup barley

1½ pounds fresh salmon, cut into 2-inch medallions

1 tablespoon extra-virgin olive oil

½ teaspoon smoked paprika

½ teaspoon salt

¼ teaspoon ground black pepper

4 cups (5 ounces) mixed greens, washed

2 cups sugar snap peas, blanched, with ends trimmed off and sliced in half so the pea inside is showing

1 medium zucchini, seeds discarded, sliced into ribbons using peeler or mandoline*

1 medium English cucumber, seeds discarded, sliced into ribbons using peeler or mandoline*

---

* If you don't want to take the time to make zucchini and cucumber ribbons, you can slice them into half-moons or strips; ribbons just make a nice presentation.

Dressing:

½ avocado

2 green onions (scallions), roughly chopped

1 tablespoon lemon juice (the juice from one lemon)

½ tablespoon fresh dill, just leaves

2 tablespoons fresh basil, chopped

2 teaspoons honey

1 clove garlic

½ cup water

Salt and pepper to taste

1. Preheat oven to 350°F; place a rimmed baking sheet in the oven.

(RECIPE CONTINUES ON NEXT PAGE)

2. Prepare the barley following the package instructions. Once cooked, allow to cool.

3. Season the salmon medallions with the olive oil, smoked paprika, salt, and pepper.

4. Oil the heated baking sheet, place the salmon medallions on it, and put it into oven until salmon is cooked through, reaching an internal temperature of 145°F, about 15 minutes. (The heated baking sheet will help crisp up the skin.)

5. While the salmon bakes, make the dressing: In a food processor or blender, combine all the ingredients and process on high until slightly thick and creamy; you can adjust consistency by adding more water.

6. In a large bowl, toss together the salad ingredients and barley with the dressing until well coated.

7. Place the salmon medallions over salad and serve family style or as individual portions.

NUTRITIONAL IMPACT PER SERVING: 39 g protein, 15 g fat, 25 g carbohydrates, 6 g fiber, 88 mg calcium, 1,039 mg potassium, 507 mg sodium, 7.06 mcg B12, 0.05 leucine, 26 mg vitamin C, 390 calories

Tips and Secrets

Make the barley ahead of time. In fact, make more than you need and keep it in your refrigerator to use in other meals during the week; add it to soup, flavor it with broth, or serve as a side dish—there are lots of options.

Fun Fact

THE BARLEY NECESSITIES: Barley comes in two different varieties: hulled and pearled. Hulled barley is higher in protein and fiber because it is unrefined. Barley contains gluten, so if you have celiac disease or a gluten sensitivity, find a substitute such as quinoa.

German Steak and Potato Salad
(Gluten-free, dairy-free)

Maybe you don't expect to see steak and potatoes in a "diet" book, but this meal is high in protein and perfect as a summertime BBQ option!

4 SERVINGS

1 cup frozen green peas

1½ pounds fingerling potatoes (4 cups), cut in half

1½ pounds flank steak, fat trimmed off

1 tablespoon extra-virgin olive oil

½ teaspoon salt

¼ teaspoon ground black pepper

1 cup (about 15 to 16) cherry tomatoes

½ red onion (1 cup), finely diced

3 cups watercress (if you can't find watercress, use arugula)

Dressing:

¼ cup apple cider vinegar or red wine vinegar

1 tablespoon extra-virgin olive oil

2 tablespoons fresh parsley, finely chopped

1 tablespoon Dijon mustard

¼ cup chives, finely chopped

½ teaspoon smoked paprika

Salt and pepper to taste

1. Preheat oven to 400°F and heat up your outdoor or indoor grill to medium-high heat.

2. Blanch the peas by dropping them into a pot of rapidly boiling water. Let them cook for just 1½ minutes. Drain quickly in a colander.

3. Cook the potatoes until they are fork tender, about 15 minutes; be sure not to overcook. Rinse under cold water to stop the cooking.

4. While the potatoes are boiling, rub the flank steak with the olive oil, salt, and pepper.

(RECIPE CONTINUES ON NEXT PAGE)

5. Place the steak on the grill and cook for about 10 minutes until it reaches an internal temperature of 135°F for medium rare or longer if you want the steak well done.

6. While the steak is cooking, place the tomatoes on a rimmed baking sheet, and roast in oven until they are blistered, 15 to 20 minutes.

7. Remove the steak from grill and let rest for 10 minutes to allow the juices to redistribute before slicing.

8. In a small bowl, combine the salad dressing ingredients and whisk well.

9. In a large bowl, combine the cooked potatoes, peas, tomatoes, onion, watercress, and dressing. Toss until all ingredients are well incorporated.

10. Serve the salad topped with sliced flank steak either family style or on individual plates.

NUTRITIONAL IMPACT PER SERVING: 42 g protein, 21 g fat, 38 g carbohydrates, 8 g fiber, 96 mg calcium, 1,534 mg potassium, 439 mg sodium, 2.01 mcg B12, 2.95 g leucine, 60 mg vitamin C, 512 calories

Tips and Secrets

Make the salad dressing and/or the potatoes ahead of time. Blanch the peas earlier in the day.

Feta Fish Fest

Another classic Mediterranean dish. You can sub out the rustic whole grain bread, using brown rice, barley, farro, whole grain pita, or any other high-fiber grain or bread instead. If you are not a fan of shrimp, you can use a meaty white fish instead, such as cod, haddock, bass, flounder, grouper, or snapper. Serve with a simple green salad.

4 SERVINGS

3 tablespoons extra-virgin olive oil, divided

1 cup shallots, finely diced

4 cloves garlic, finely chopped or grated

1 pound chopped tomatoes (canned, unsalted)

1 teaspoon tomato paste

Salt and pepper to taste

1 teaspoon crushed red pepper flakes

½ teaspoon dried oregano

Juice and zest of 1 lemon

¼ cup kalamata olives (about 16 olives), pitted and cut in half

1 pound large shrimp (about 28), peeled and deveined

¾ cup Greek feta cheese, crumbled

¼ cup panko bread crumbs

1 tablespoon parsley (for garnish)

4 slices (1-inch-thick) artisan whole grain bread, toasted

1. Preheat oven to 375°F.

2. Heat a cast-iron pan over medium heat. (If you don't have cast iron, you can use any shallow pan and then transfer to a baking dish before throwing into the oven.)

3. When the pan is too hot to touch, heat 1 tablespoon of the olive oil. Sauté the shallots until translucent, then add the garlic and sauté about 1 minute more.

4. Add the tomatoes and tomato paste and stir well. Bring to a boil and then reduce to a simmer for 2 to 3 minutes for sauce to thicken.

5. Add the salt, pepper, red pepper flakes, oregano, lemon juice, lemon zest, and olives. Stir well and simmer for another 2 to 3 minutes.

(RECIPE CONTINUES ON NEXT PAGE)

6. Add the shrimp, evenly dispersing in the pan for even cooking. Top the shrimp and sauce with the crumbled feta and bread crumbs and drizzle with the remaining 2 tablespoons of olive oil.

7. Place the cast-iron pan in oven and bake 10 to 15 minutes or until the shrimp are cooked and the panko is golden and crunchy.

8. Sprinkle with the parsley and serve family style in the skillet with toasted bread on the side for dipping.

NUTRTIONAL IMPACT PER SERVING: 26 g protein, 23 g fat, 39 g carbohydrates, 7 g fiber, 490 mg calcium, 636 mg potassium, 1,406 mg sodium, 1.74 mcg B12, 1.73 g leucine, 29 mg vitamin C, 466 calories

Turkey Stuffed and Squashed
(Gluten-free, dairy-free)

This is a complete meal on its own, but it never hurts to have additional vegetables, so feel free to serve it with a simple side salad. Enjoy a nice cup of fresh berries for dessert to increase fiber.

4 SERVINGS

2 medium acorn squash, ends sliced off, sliced in half widthwise, seeds scooped out

2 tablespoons extra-virgin olive oil, divided

1 tablespoon maple syrup

Filling:

1 medium carrot, peeled and roughly chopped (½ cup)

8 medium button or Baby Bella mushrooms, cut in half

1 shallot, roughly chopped (½ cup)

2 tablespoons basil

3 cloves garlic

1 pound ground turkey

1 cup cooked brown rice (follow cooking instructions on package)

Salt and pepper to taste

1 package (5 ounces) baby kale, chopped

1. Preheat oven to 400°F.

2. Place the acorn squash halves flesh side up in a shallow baking dish. Rub each half with 1 tablespoon of the olive oil and maple syrup.

3. Bake the squash for 40 to 45 minutes until tender.

4. While the squash is baking, make the filling: In a food processor, combine the carrots, mushrooms, shallot, basil, and garlic in a food processor and process on high until vegetables are finely chopped (not pureed).

(RECIPE CONTINUES ON NEXT PAGE)

5. In a large skillet, heat remaining 1 tablespoon of the olive oil over medium heat. Add the veggie mixture and sauté 2 to 3 minutes.

6. Add ground turkey to the mixture and continue to sauté until turkey is fully cooked.

7. Add the brown rice, salt, and pepper.

8. When all the ingredients are well incorporated, add the baby kale and cook until it has wilted.

9. Divide the mixture evenly among the four cooked squash "bowls." Place back into oven for 5 to 10 minutes before serving.

NUTRITIONAL IMPACT PER SERVING: 36 g protein, 19 g fat, 46 g carbohydrates, 6 g fiber, 156 mg calcium, 1,342 mg potassium, 580 mg sodium, 1.51 mcg B12, 0.14 g leucine, 51 mg vitamin C, 485 calories

RECIPE VARIATION
You can add grated Parmesan on top before baking for a nice crispy and cheesy topping.

Fun Fact

TAP INTO THIS: Yes, maple syrup is a form of sugar, but it provides (albeit negligible) nutrients, including calcium and zinc, compared to highly processed corn-syrup-laden pancake syrup, which has none.

So Farro, So Good Chicken with Bok Choy

(Dairy-free)

A nutrient-dense grain, farro makes a nice change from rice. This complete meal uses it as a base to mix up the standard chicken-and-rice dish, and adds in bok choy, a cruciferous vegetable packed with vitamins A and C.

4 SERVINGS

Chicken:

1 pound thin chicken breast sliced into strips

¼ cup teriyaki sauce

Fried Farro:

2 teaspoons extra virgin olive oil

½ medium onion, chopped

1½ medium carrots, diced into small cubes (¾ cup)

¾ cup frozen peas

2 eggs

1 cup cooked farro (follow instructions on packet; a 10-minute variety is fine)

1 tablespoon reduced-sodium soy sauce

Bok Choy:

1 teaspoon extra-virgin olive oil

2 cloves garlic, thinly sliced

1 teaspoon fresh ginger, finely chopped or grated

1 pound baby bok choy, sliced in half, stem ends cut off (may seem like a lot, but bok choy wilts)

Salt and pepper to taste

1. Marinate the chicken breast in teriyaki sauce for 20 to 60 minutes.

2. While the chicken is marinating, make the fried farro: In a pan or wok, heat the olive oil over medium heat. When the oil is hot, sauté the onions and the carrots until the onions are translucent and the carrots have softened a bit, about 5 minutes. Add the frozen peas and cook until they are heated through.

(RECIPE CONTINUES ON NEXT PAGE)

3. Make a well in the middle of the sautéed veggies, crack the eggs into it, and let them fry for about 1 minute. When the whites have turned from clear to white, begin scrambling the yolk. Incorporate the scrambled eggs into sautéed veggies.

4. Add the cooked farro and mix well until heated through. Add the soy sauce and stir well. Keep the heat on medium 1 to 2 minutes to allow the farro to crisp up a bit.

5. Remove the farro and plate. Cover with foil or place in oven-safe dish and put in the oven to keep warm while you make the chicken and bok choy.

6. For the bok choy: In a pan or wok (use the same one in which you cooked the farro), heat the olive oil over medium heat. Sauté the garlic and ginger about 30 seconds. Add the bok choy and sauté until it has wilted but is still al dente. Season with salt and pepper. Set bok choy aside.

7. Using the same hot pan used for the bok choy, cook the chicken with the marinade over medium heat 7 to 8 minutes, stirring occasionally, until chicken is fully cooked and has reached an internal temperature of 165°F.

8. Serve either family style or plated individually.

NUTRITIONAL IMPACT PER SERVING: 36 g protein, 8 g fat, 24 g carbohydrates, 5 g fiber, 149 mg calcium, 265 mg potassium, 1,057 mg sodium, 0.22 mcg B12, 0.38 g leucine, 54 mg vitamin C, 309 calories

RECIPE VARIATIONS
In place of the chicken, substitute fish or beef or a vegetarian option such as tofu or tempeh.

Tips and Secrets

Make the farro ahead of time so it is as easy as pulling it from the refrigerator.

Stone-Cold Soba Noodles

(Gluten-free, dairy-free, vegetarian)

This soba noodle recipe uses peanut butter for flavor and tofu for protein. Tofu has a distinct texture and easily takes on the flavor of the sauce or marinade it is prepared with. If you prefer, you can substitute any protein such as tempeh, shrimp, scallops, chicken, beef, pork, or fish. All would work in this delicious noodle dish.

4 SERVINGS

Cooking oil spray
12 ounces extra-firm tofu, cut into ½ inch cubes

Peanut sauce:

¼ cup creamy peanut butter
2 tablespoons reduced-sodium soy sauce, (if you're gluten free, be sure to use gluten-free soy sauce)
2 tablespoons red wine vinegar
1 tablespoon sesame oil

1 tablespoon cilantro, finely chopped
1 tablespoon honey
1 tablespoon sambal, a spicy sauce made from chile peppers and garlic (optional)

Noodles:

4½ ounces dried 100% buckwheat soba noodles, cooked (following package instructions) and cooled
2 Persian cucumbers*, julienned (1 cup)
1 medium carrot, julienned (¾ cup)
5 green onions, thinly sliced
1 cup edamame, fully cooked and shelled

1 medium red bell pepper, thinly sliced
1 tablespoon minced jalapeño pepper (optional)
⅓ cup cilantro, roughly chopped (for garnish)
2 tablespoons peanuts, crushed (for garnish)

---

* Persian cucumbers are thin and have ridges; most large markets carry them.

(RECIPE CONTINUES ON NEXT PAGE)

1. Coat a medium skillet with the cooking oil spray. Sauté the tofu over medium heat until all sides are browned.

2. In a small bowl, whisk together all the ingredients for peanut sauce until creamy.

3. In a large bowl, toss together all the ingredients for the noodles except the cilantro and crushed peanuts. Add the tofu.

4. Add the peanut sauce to the noodle/tofu mixture and toss until all the ingredients are well coated.

5. Garnish with cilantro and crushed peanuts, and serve family style or as individual portions.

NUTRITIONAL IMPACT PER SERVING: 25 g protein, 22 g fat, 43 g carbohydrates, 6 g fiber, 217 mg calcium, 574 mg potassium, 480 mg sodium, 0 mcg B12, 0.1 g leucine, 56 mg vitamin C, 456 calories

Steak à la Chimichurri, Chimichurri, Chimichurri Churri!

(Gluten-free, dairy-free)

By serving this steak dish with a high-fiber grain or starch such as brown rice, farro, barley, or lentils, while pairing with grilled or roasted vegetables such as asparagus, broccoli, zucchini, or brussels sprouts, you will bring the fiber up to the Whole Body Reset standards. Soak the wood skewers in water for at least 30 minutes.

4 SERVINGS

Steak:

- 1½ pounds filet mignon or sirloin, cut into 2-inch cubes
- 3 cloves garlic (1 tablespoon), finely chopped
- ½ teaspoon salt
- ¼ teaspoon ground black pepper
- ½ medium yellow onion, cut into 2-inch chunks
- 1 medium orange bell pepper, cut into 2-inch chunks
- 8 Baby Bella or button mushrooms, left whole with steams removed

Chimichurri sauce:

- ½ cup cilantro
- ½ cup parsley
- 3 cloves garlic
- ¼ teaspoon salt
- ¼ teaspoon ground black pepper
- ¼ teaspoon crushed red pepper flakes
- 1 tablespoon water
- 4 teaspoons apple cider vinegar
- 2 tablespoons extra-virgin olive oil

1. For the steak: Rub the steak cubes with garlic, salt, and pepper and allow to marinate for 20 minutes.

2. If grilling the meat, fire up outdoor grill or turn on an indoor grill to medium; if roasting, preheat oven to 350°F.

(RECIPE CONTINUES ON NEXT PAGE)

3. Make the chimichurri sauce: In a food processor, combine all the ingredients except the olive oil and pulse a few times for a rough chop.

4. While the food processor is still on, slowly drizzle in the olive oil. Process until the ingredients are finely minced. You can also puree for a smoother sauce.

5. Assemble the skewers, placing one cube of steak, a chunk of onion, a chunk of pepper, and a whole mushroom, and so on until there are three cubes of steak on each skewer.

6. Place the kebobs on grill or in oven, turning every 4 to 5 minutes until all sides are nicely browned and caramelized.

7. Plate the kabobs on platter and drizzle chimichurri sauce over them before serving.

NUTRITIONAL IMPACT PER SERVING: 40 g protein, 19 g fat, 8 g carbohydrates, 2 g fiber, 81 mg calcium, 849 mg potassium, 543 mg sodium, 2.05 mcg B12, 3.07 g leucine, 60 mg vitamin C, 369 calories

Tips and Secrets

You can find precut raw grilling vegetables (onions, peppers, zucchini, mushrooms, asparagus) in the produce section in many supermarkets, often on skewers. You can even find steak or chicken kebobs already prepared, either unseasoned or with store-made marinade.

Fun Fact

MOUTH WASH? Some people describe the taste of cilantro as "soapy." This taste sensation is actually genetic! If you inherited the anti-cilantro gene, try substituting parsley, which is in the same family, in your recipe.

A Chicken in Every Pot

(Gluten-free, dairy-free)

This one-pot meal incorporates split peas, a member of the legume family that provides protein, fiber, potassium, magnesium, and iron. Since the peas are split, they cook faster, eliminating the need to presoak. Simply sort and rinse before cooking. If you do not want to cook the peas, look for canned yellow peas (usually in the international foods aisle), lentils, or pigeon peas. Just rinse before using to wash away the sodium.

4 SERVINGS

2 tablespoons extra-virgin olive oil

1 large red bell pepper, diced (1 cup)

4 cloves garlic, thinly sliced (about 1½ tablespoons)

1 medium sweet onion, diced (1¾ cups)

2 medium carrots, chopped (1 cup)

1 tablespoon fresh ginger, grated or finely chopped

2 tablespoons ground turmeric

½ tablespoon crushed red pepper flakes

2 tablespoons ground cumin

1 tablespoon smoked paprika

4 boneless, skinless chicken thighs (1½ pounds)

Salt and pepper to taste

1 cup yellow split peas

4 cups low-sodium chicken broth

1 tablespoon fresh cilantro, chopped (for garnish)

1. In a large pan, heat the olive oil over medium heat and sauté the bell pepper, garlic, onion, carrots, and ginger for 5 minutes, stirring occasionally.

2. Add the turmeric, red pepper flakes, cumin, and paprika and stir together well. Cook on medium heat for 1 to 2 minutes while stirring constantly so that the spices cook but do not burn. (Toasting the spices brings out the natural oils, which gives the dish more aroma.)

(RECIPE CONTINUES ON NEXT PAGE)

3. Season the chicken with salt and pepper.

4. Add the chicken to pan, cook for 5 minutes, then turn. (The chicken will have plenty of time to cook while simmering in the sauce.)

5. Pour the yellow peas into the pan and give a quick stir to evenly combine.

6. Add the chicken broth to the pan and bring to a boil. Allow to boil for 2 minutes, then reduce to a simmer, cover pan, and simmer for 40 minutes to an hour. Check about halfway through. If the sauce is thick, add more chicken broth or water.

7. When the peas are fully cooked, season with salt and pepper to taste. Garnish with the cilantro. Serve family style.

NUTRITIONAL IMPACT PER SERVING: 32 g protein, 13 g fat, 52 g carbohydrates, 17 g fiber, 90 mg calcium, 1,126 mg potassium, 169 mg sodium, 0.24 mcg B12, 0.1 g leucine, 55 mg vitamin C, 441 calories

What's Shakin' Shakshuka

(Gluten-free)

Besides being fun to pronounce, this shakshuka makes for a flavor-packed brunch, and it's high in protein and fiber, too. It can be served with a multigrain pita or a slice of whole grain artisan bread for dipping. If you do not want to create shakshuka sauce from scratch, you may find it already made in the same aisle you find olives and roasted red peppers.

4 SERVINGS

2 tablespoons extra-virgin olive oil

½ sweet onion (¾ cup), finely diced

3 cloves garlic, minced or grated

½ red bell pepper (½ cup), finely diced

¼ cup uncooked quinoa, rinsed

Salt and pepper to taste

½ teaspoon red pepper flakes

½ teaspoon smoked paprika

1 can (15½ ounces) chickpeas (garbanzos), drained and rinsed

1 can (15 ounces) crushed tomatoes

½ cup chicken broth

1 cup (15 to 16) fresh cherry tomatoes

8 large eggs

5 ounces (about ½ cup) plain nonfat Greek yogurt

Juice (½ tablespoon) and zest from ½ lemon

1 tablespoon cilantro, roughly chopped (for garnish)

2 tablespoon chives, finely chopped (for garnish)

1. In a large cast-iron skillet or shallow pan, heat the olive oil over medium heat. When oil is hot, add the onion, garlic, and bell pepper and sauté for 5 to 6 minutes until tender, stirring occasionally.

2. Add the quinoa to the pan and cook for 2 minutes, stirring occasionally. Add salt, pepper, red pepper flakes, and paprika.

3. Add in the chickpeas, crushed tomatoes, and chicken broth. Bring to a boil for 1 minute, then reduce to a simmer on low heat

(RECIPE CONTINUES ON NEXT PAGE)

and cook 35 to 40 minutes or until quinoa is cooked, stirring occasionally. Cover pan halfway through. If sauce becomes too thick, add a bit more chicken broth to thin it out (start with ⅓ cup).

4. While the quinoa mixture cooks, preheat oven to 375°F.

5. Place the cherry tomatoes on a rimmed baking sheet and roast until tomatoes are blistered, about 5 minutes.

6. When the quinoa is done cooking, make 4 small pockets in the mixture and crack the eggs into them. Place skillet in oven and bake for 5 to 7 minutes or until yolks are to desired doneness.

7. While the eggs are cooking, make the yogurt sauce by whisking together the yogurt, lemon juice, and zest.

8. Remove the quinoa from the oven. Toss the roasted tomatoes on top, garnish with the cilantro and chives, and dollop a few spoonfuls of the yogurt sauce around the skillet.

NUTRITIONAL IMPACT PER SERVING: 25 g protein, 19 g fat, 38 g carbohydrates, 9 g fiber, 206 mg calcium, 1,066 mg potassium, 654 mg sodium, 1.16 mcg B12, 0.43 g leucine, 51 mg vitamin C, 410 calories

Tips and Secrets

To shorten the cooking time, you can also use frozen cooked quinoa that can be found in most large grocery stores.

Soups, Salads, and Sides

These recipes aren't complete meals—meaning they won't deliver all the protein and fiber you need at any given mealtime. Consider them more like upgrades for any simply prepared (grilled, roasted, broiled) main-dish protein you make. Plus, each offers an additional boost of protein and fiber, so they can help top off your tank at snack time, especially if you'd prefer a smaller portion of one of our complete meals.

Can't Lose Couscous Soup
(Dairy-free)

4 SERVINGS

1 tablespoon extra-virgin olive oil or avocado oil

4 cups (1¼ pounds) butternut squash, diced into ½-inch cubes

1 small white onion, diced

3 large cloves garlic, thinly sliced

5 cups low-sodium chicken broth

1 teaspoon sea salt, or to taste

1 cup dry whole wheat couscous

1 package (5 ounces) baby kale, chopped

1. In a large saucepan, heat the olive oil over medium-high heat. Add the squash and onion and cook while stirring until the onion is fully softened, about 8 minutes.

2. Add the garlic and cook while stirring until fragrant, about 1 minute.

3. Add the broth and salt and bring to a boil over high heat. Reduce heat to medium and cook, uncovered, until the squash is just tender, about 5 minutes.

4. Reduce heat to low, stir in the couscous and kale, and cook uncovered until couscous is cooked through, about 5 minutes more.

5. Adjust seasoning and serve.

NUTRITIONAL IMPACT PER SERVING: 11 g protein, 6 g fat, 38 g carbohydrates, 6 g fiber, 152 mg calcium, 1,029 mg potassium, 704 mg sodium, 0.3 mcg B12, 0.1 g leucine, 76 mg vitamin C, 230 calories

Ginger Spice Bisque

(Gluten-free, with vegetarian and vegan alternatives)

It's posh, too. Serve it hot or cold for a nice dose of Vitamin A!

6 SERVINGS

Coconut oil cooking spray
1 cup onion, diced
1 tablespoon peeled ginger,
   minced
2 cups low-sodium chicken
   broth or vegetable broth
1 pound carrots, peeled and
   cut into chunks plus ¼ cup
   carrot shavings for garnish

2 large unpeeled pears, diced
1 bay leaf
1½ cups nonfat half-and-half,
   or dairy-free almond or
   coconut low-fat creamer
Salt and pepper to taste
¼ cup dill for garnish

1. In a large saucepan sprayed with cooking spray, sauté the onion over medium heat until translucent and tender.

2. Add the ginger and sauté another minute or two.

3. Add the chicken broth, carrot chunks, pears, and bay leaf, and simmer, partly covered, until the carrots are tender.

4. Remove the bay leaf. In a blender or food processor, puree the mixture blending in the half-and-half to thin the soup to your taste. Season with salt and pepper.

5. Reheat the soup gently, and serve it hot, or let it cool completely, place in refrigerator for 2 hours, and serve cold with a garnish of carrot shavings and fresh dill.

NUTRITIONAL IMPACT PER SERVING: 5 g protein, 2 g fat, 30 g carbohydrates, 5 g fiber, 104 mg calcium, 598 mg potassium, 142 mg sodium, 0.39 mcg B12, 0.07 g leucine, 11 mg vitamin C, 146 calories

Fun Fact

GINGER-VITIS: Ginger is well known for its ability to soothe an upset stomach and nausea but is also good for oral health. The compound gingerol helps fight oral bacteria and keep your mouth fresh and clean.

Bill's Maryland Crab Soup
(Gluten-free)

Bill Hawkins, on our Whole Body Reset test panel, used this recipe to help fuel his workouts. During the COVID lockdown, this soup was part of his the Whole Body Reset regimen. Make this a complete meal by serving it with a fruit salad or whole fruit to up your fiber.

10 SERVINGS

2 quarts chicken or beef stock (Bill uses a combination of 1 quart each)

3 pounds diced canned tomatoes, with juice

1½ cups celery, sliced

1½ cups yellow onion, shredded

⅓ cup carrot, diced

¾ cups green bell pepper, diced

½ cup butter

2 cups tomato puree

4 to 6 tablespoons Old Bay Seasoning

⅛ teaspoon salt

¼ teaspoon black pepper

1 to 2 pounds lump crabmeat

1. In a large pot, combine the stock and diced tomatoes over medium-high heat.

2. Add the celery, onion, carrot, green pepper, and butter.

3. Blend in the tomato puree.

4. Add the Old Bay, salt, and pepper.

5. Bring to low boil, reduce the heat to low, cover, and simmer for 1 hour.

6. Add the crabmeat.

7. Cook for about 10 minutes more and serve.

NUTRITIONAL IMPACT PER SERVING. 10 g protein, 10 g fat, 17 g carbohydrates, 4 g fiber, 168 mg calcium, 643 mg potassium, 2,336 mg sodium, 0.02 mcg B12, 0.04 g leucine, 27 g vitamin C, 239 calories

Caribbean Vacation Chicken Soup

(Gluten-free, dairy-free)

On a cold day, cook up this vegetable-packed stew, crank up the Wailers, close your eyes, and pretend you're lolling on a seaside hammock, knowing that the high fiber and protein content is getting you closer to that dream swimsuit. Mojito not included.

6 SERVINGS

2 medium carrots, chopped

2 medium celery stalks, diced

1 red bell pepper, chopped into large pieces

½ yellow onion, chopped

3 cloves garlic, roughly chopped

½ small calabaza (pumpkin) or squash, diced

½ sweet potato, chopped into half-moon quarter-inch pieces

1 semi-ripe plantain, sliced

1 cup low-sodium canned black beans, drained and rinsed

4 cups low-sodium chicken broth

Kosher or sea salt to taste

Black pepper to taste

3 skinless, boneless chicken breasts

1 teaspoon olive oil or chili/garlic oil

1 handful (about 1 cup) spinach

½ bunch of cilantro (cut off bottom stems)

1. In a large pot, heat the vegetables (except the spinach and cilantro) and chicken broth over high heat.

2. Bring to a boil for 15 minutes, then reduce to medium-low heat.

3. Sprinkle salt and pepper on both sides of the chicken breasts.

4. In a sauté pan, heat the olive oil and sear the chicken on both sides until browned.

5. Remove the chicken from the pan, cut into pieces, and add to soup. Cook for 30 minutes.

6. In a food processor or blender, puree the spinach, cilantro, and a cup of the soup.

7. Incorporate the puree into the remaining soup; cook 15 more minutes.

8. Add salt and pepper to taste.

NUTRITIONAL IMPACT PER SERVING: 23 g protein, 3 g fat, 29 g carbohydrates, 6 g fiber, 62 mg calcium, 1,028 mg potassium, 184 mg sodium, 0.12 mcg B12, 1.38 g leucine, 49 mg vitamin C, 231 calories

VARIATIONS
You can use all pumpkin, all squash, or all sweet potato, but variety lends textures, flavors, and nutrition.

Totally Nutty Sweet Potatoes
(Gluten-free, dairy-free, vegetarian)

A perfect side dish to add fiber and flavor. Serve with a protein such as turkey breast or turkey burger for a complete meal. Also makes a great side dish for Thanksgiving!

4 SERVINGS

Sweet Potatoes:

3 large sweet potatoes (1½ pounds), cubed (keep skin on for more vitamins and minerals)

1 tablespoon extra-virgin olive oil
½ teaspoon coconut oil
1 teaspoon ground cinnamon
¼ teaspoon ground nutmeg

Dressing:

Juice and zest from 1 orange (2 tablespoons)
Juice and zest from 1 lemon (1 tablespoon)
½ teaspoon fresh ginger, grated or finely chopped

2 tablespoons honey
1 tablespoon extra-virgin olive oil
½ tablespoon red wine vinegar
Salt and pepper to taste

Garnish:

2 tablespoons hazelnuts, crushed

¼ cup fresh pomegranate seeds

1. Preheat oven to 400°F.

2. Place the sweet potato cubes on a rimmed baking sheet.

3. In a small bowl, combine the olive oil, coconut oil, cinnamon, and nutmeg and mix well. Pour over sweet potatoes and toss.

4. Bake the sweet potatoes for 20 to 30 minutes until potatoes are fork tender, not mushy.

5. While the sweet potatoes bake, make the dressing: In a small bowl, whisk together all the ingredients.

6. In a large bowl, combine the sweet potatoes and dressing and toss well. (The sweet potatoes should absorb most of the dressing.)

7. Plate the sweet potatoes on a platter, discarding remaining dressing. Top with the crushed hazelnuts and pomegranate seeds.

NUTRITIONAL IMPACT PER SERVING: 2 g protein, 10 g fat, 33 g carbohydrates, 4 g fiber, 43 mg calcium, 409 mg potassium, 56 mg sodium, 0 mcg B12, 0.13 g leucine, 8 mg vitamin C, 219 calories

Fun Fact

FIRE FIGHTER: Cinnamon reduces inflammation by blocking your body's release of an inflammatory compound called arachidonic acid. Sprinkle this tasty spice on everything from toast to apples and mix into baked items as well as savory stews.

Crèmes and Misdemeanors
(Gluten-free, dairy-free, vegetarian, vegan)

This walnut crème adds a smooth panache to any green vegetable or even roasted carrots or sweet potatoes. Feel free to substitute the broccolini with regular broccoli, asparagus, broccoli rabe, or sautéed spinach. To make a complete meal and up the fiber, serve with grilled fish, chicken, or tofu, and brown rice or baked potato.

Remember to leave time for the walnuts to soak.

4 SERVINGS

Walnut crème:

½ cup walnuts, raw, unsalted
½ teaspoon salt
⅛ teaspoon ground black
  pepper

2 cloves garlic
½ cup water

Broccolini:

½ teaspoon salt
14 ounces broccolini (about
  5½ cups), with stem ends
  trimmed off

1 tablespoon walnuts, raw,
  unsalted, crushed
Salt and pepper to taste

1. Make the walnut crème: Soak the walnuts, salt, pepper, and garlic in water for at least 2 hours; soaking overnight is best.

2. Place all walnut crème ingredients in a blender and blend on high until smooth and creamy. Set aside.

3. To eliminate the raw taste of the walnuts, pour the walnut crème into a small pot over medium heat and heat through. (The walnut crème raw, without cooking, is also delicious.)

4. Make the broccolini: In a large pot, bring 4 cups of salted water to a boil. Add broccolini and cook for 3 minutes; it should be bright green and al dente.

5. Plate the broccolini on a platter, pour the walnut crème over the top of the stems, and sprinkle with the crushed walnuts.

6. Add salt and pepper to taste, and serve.

NUTRITIONAL IMPACT PER SERVING: 6 g protein, 15 g fat, 6 g carbohydrate, 4 g fiber, 127 mg calcium, 267 mg potassium, 905 mg sodium, 0 mcg B12, 0.34 g leucine, 21 mg vitamin C, 163 calories

Hustled-Up Brussels Salad with Green Apple Dressing
(Gluten-free, vegetarian)

Add grilled shrimp, chicken, fish, or hard-boiled eggs to increase the protein and make this a complete meal instead of a side dish. If you cannot find tart cherries, use any dried fruit such as raisins, dried cranberries, or dried blueberries. You can also substitute pumpkin seeds with sunflower seeds or slivered almonds.

4 SERVINGS

Salad:

4½ cups brussels sprouts, shredded

2 cups coleslaw mix (red and white cabbage with shredded carrots)

¾ cup roasted pumpkin seeds (pepitas), unsalted

½ cup tart cherries, dried and pitted

½ cup Parmesan cheese, shaved

Dressing:

1 medium green apple, peeled, cored, and cut into cubes

2 tablespoons extra-virgin olive oil

1 teaspoon Dijon mustard

3 tablespoons apple cider vinegar

2 tablespoons honey

1 tablespoon water

Salt and pepper to taste

1. In a large bowl, combine all the salad ingredients.

2. Combine all the dressing ingredients in a blender and blend on high until smooth, making sure the apple is pureed very well.

3. Toss the salad with dressing and serve.

NUTRITIONAL IMPACT PER SERVING: 14 g protein, 21 g fat, 42 g carbohydrates, 7 g fiber, 158 mg calcium, 640 mg potassium, 232 mg sodium, 0.14 mcg B12, 0.89 g leucine, 96 mg vitamin C, 381 calories

Can't Be Beet Citrus Salad

(Gluten-free, vegetarian)

A refreshing and colorful side salad. Pair with your favorite protein and whole grain starch to make this a tasty and light meal. This salad will add a tropical tang alongside a simple grilled white fish or baked chicken, and quinoa adds a nice texture, as well as protein.

4 SERVINGS

1 pound prepared beets, cut into chunks

1 ruby red grapefruit, segmented (¾ cup)

1 pink grapefruit, segmented (1 cup)

1 medium orange, segmented (¾ cup)

2 tablespoons unsalted pistachios, roasted and ground

¼ cup soft goat cheese, crumbled

1 teaspoon fresh mint, chopped

Dressing:

½ tablespoon chopped shallot (½ shallot)

1 tablespoon red wine vinegar

½ tablespoon orange juice

½ tablespoon extra-virgin olive oil

1 tablespoon honey (or date syrup, agave, or another sweetener)

Salt and pepper to taste

1. Preheat oven to 375°F.

2. Place the beets on a baking sheet and roast for 10 to 15 minutes.

3. While the beets are roasting, combine all the dressing ingredients in a food processor or blender and process on high until dressing is smooth and shallots are completely pureed.

4. When the beets are done, let them cool and then toss them in a medium bowl with the dressing.

5. Plate the beets on a platter. Assemble the citrus around and on top of beets for a contrast of colors.

6. Sprinkle with the pistachios, crumbled goat cheese, and mint.

NUTRITIONAL IMPACT PER SERVING: 5 g protein, 6 g fat, 34 g carbohydrates, 6 g fiber, 101 mg calcium, 146 mg potassium, 94 mg sodium, 0.02 mcg B12, 0.01 g leucine, 72 mg vitamin C, 207 calories

Tips and Secrets

- You can find prepared beets in the refrigerated produce section. Or prepare your own, getting raw beets from the produce department and then removing the tops and the taproots (on the bottom) and peeling with a vegetable peeler. Cut the beets into 1½-inch chunks. Place the cut beets on a rimmed baking sheet and toss with olive oil, salt, and pepper. Roast for 35 to 40 minutes, turning once or twice with a spatula, until the beets are tender.

- If you would like to get more creative with this dish, you can roll the goat cheese into little balls and coat them in the ground pistachio.

- Feel free to use any type of citrus you would like. If you do not like grapefruit, try an array of oranges such as cara cara, navel, and blood.

Fun Fact

HIDE THE EVIDENCE: If beet juice gets on your hands, try rubbing lemon and salt on your hands before washing them.

Garlic and Shallot Spinach with "Yes, Please" Cheese Crisps

(Gluten-free, vegetarian)

A light and satisfying side dish. Pair with steak and a baked potato to feel like you are enjoying a nice but healthy steakhouse dinner. Not a fan of steak? This vegetable dish will pair nicely with any protein and starch.

4 SERVINGS

4 tablespoons grated pecorino cheese (or its close cousin, Parmesan)

2 tablespoons extra-virgin olive oil

2 shallots thinly sliced (about 1 cup)

4 cloves garlic

18 ounces fresh spinach

Salt and pepper to taste

1. Preheat oven to 375°F.

2. On a greased baking sheet, make pecorino crisps by measuring ½ tablespoon of the cheese into flat circles (like pancakes). This should make 8 circles.

3. Bake the crisps for 3 to 5 minutes (watch carefully, they cook fast). When the cheese is browned, remove from the oven and allow to rest to become crisp.

4. In a shallow pan, heat the olive oil over medium heat. Sauté the shallots until translucent, then add the garlic to pan and sauté about 1 minute more.

5. Slowly add and wilt the spinach; add more spinach as it wilts.

6. Plate the sautéed spinach with shallots and garlic on a platter, top with the pecorino crisps, add salt and pepper, and serve.

NUTRITIONAL IMPACT PER SERVING: 8 g protein, 10 g fat, 9 g carbohydrates, 4 g fiber, 283 mg calcium, 789 mg potassium, 274 mg sodium, 0 mcg B12, 0.04 g leucine, 39 mg vitamin C, 164 calories

Tips and Secrets

Pecorino cheese is very salty and becomes saltier as it bakes, so you may not want to add salt until you have tasted the finished dish.

Make extra pecorino cheese crisps and have them as a snack or with a salad to provide some crunch and flavor.

Farm Stand Salad with Roasted Garlic Dressing

(Gluten-free, dairy-free, vegetarian)

A salad full of color, textures, and flavor, pulled from whatever's in season at your local farm stand. It is low-calorie and light, a perfect accompaniment to serve with grilled lamb chops and brown basmati rice, or any protein and grain of choice.

4 SERVINGS

1 medium zucchini, sliced in half lengthwise and into half-moons (about 2 cups)

1 medium yellow squash, sliced in half lenthwise and into half-moons (about 2 cups)

1 large red onion, cut into rings (1¼ cups)

1 medium red bell pepper, cut into thick slices

12 asparagus spears, ends trimmed off, cut in half

1 cup cherry tomatoes

2 tablespoons extra-virgin olive oil

Salt and pepper to taste

1 head romaine lettuce, chopped

Dressing:

8 cloves garlic, unpeeled, tops sliced off

1½ tablespoons extra-virgin olive oil, divided

1 tablespoon Dijon mustard

1 tablespoon honey

3 tablespoons balsamic vinegar

¼ teaspoon dried thyme

½ teaspoon dried oregano

Salt and pepper to taste

1. Preheat oven to 375°F.

2. In a large bowl, toss all the cut-up vegetables except romaine lettuce with the olive oil and season with salt and pepper. Place the oiled vegetables onto a rimmed baking sheet and roast for 30 to 35 minutes or until all vegetables are cooked through, slightly browned, and al dente.

(RECIPE CONTINUES ON NEXT PAGE)

3. For the dressing: Place the garlic with ½ tablespoon of the olive oil, salt, and pepper in aluminum foil. Fold the foil to create a packet, and bake for 30 to 40 minutes, until all cloves are soft and brown. When cool, squeeze the roasted garlic from their skins; discard skin.

4. In a food processor, combine the roasted garlic, the remaining 1 tablespoon olive oil, mustard, honey, balsamic vinegar, thyme, and oregano and process on high until dressing is smooth. If the dressing is too thick, add 1 tablespoon of water to thin. Season with salt and pepper to taste. Set aside.

5. When the vegetables are cooked, take out of the oven and allow to cool slightly. Place the romaine lettuce in a bowl and top with the grilled vegetables. Pour the dressing over and mix well.

NUTRITIONAL IMPACT PER SERVING: 6 g protein, 11 g fat, 30 g carbohydrates, 8 g fiber, 120 mg calcium, 1,105 mg potassium, 69 mg sodium, 0 mcg B12, 0.18 g leucine, 95 mg vitamin C, 228 calories

Tips and Secrets

Buying precut raw grilling vegetables (onions, peppers, zucchini, mushrooms, asparagus), available from the produce section in many supermarkets, can help cut down some time and prep in this recipe.

Avocado and Tomato "Dip in the Road" Salsa

(Gluten-free, dairy-free, vegetarian, vegan)

Use this salsa as a dip with fresh jicama, carrot, or cucumber sticks; to scoop with baked fat-free tostadas; or to top your vegetable salad, taco, tamale, or fish dish.

8 SERVINGS

2 large fresh tomatoes, peeled, seeded, and chopped (see instructions below)

½ serrano or poblano (milder) pepper, or ¼ teaspoon ground chili pepper

2 avocados, 1 mashed and 1 chopped into ¼-inch chunks

2 tomatillos, chopped (or substitute green tomatoes or green bell pepper)

1 teaspoon garlic, minced

¼ small red onion, finely chopped

1 tablespoon lime juice

¼ cup fresh strawberries, chopped

Salt

Ground black pepper

⅓ cup cilantro, finely chopped

1. Prepare tomatoes: Score each tomato with an X on the bottom. Gently lower into a large pot of boiling water for 30 seconds, remove immediately, and place into a medium bowl of ice water. The peel will come right off; seeds can also be easily removed. Coarsely chop the peeled, seeded tomatoes.

2. With gloves, remove the stem from the serrano pepper, slit it, and scrape out the seeds with a small sharp knife. Chop the flesh finely.

3. In a medium bowl, combine the serrano pepper, the tomatoes, avocados, tomatillos, garlic, onion, and lime juice. Without crushing the chopped avocado, mix until well blended.

(RECIPE CONTINUES ON NEXT PAGE)

4. Delicately blend in strawberries.

5. Just before serving, add salt, pepper, and cilantro to taste.

NUTRITIONAL IMPACT PER SERVING: 2 g protein, 8 g fat, 7 g carbohydrates, 4 g fiber, 13 mg calcium, 391 mg potassium, 6 mg sodium, 0 mcg B12, 0.09 g leucine, 16 mg vitamin C, 96 calories

Jicama-Lama Salsa

(Gluten-free, dairy-free, vegetarian, vegan)

This salsa can be used as a dressing for a green salad, as a topping for nachos or tacos, or on top of grilled fish or baked ham.

4 SERVINGS

1 small red onion, finely diced

Juice of 2 key limes (or use regular limes or ¼ cup bottled lime juice)

3 mandarin orange sections, diced; use canned mandarin oranges and reserve about 2 tablespoons of juice

2 cups jicama, peeled, cut into quarters, rinsed in cold water, and diced

1 cucumber, sliced in half lengthwise, seeds scooped out, and sliced into half-moons

1 serrano or poblano (milder) pepper), or ¼ teaspoon ground chili pepper

1. In a small bowl, combine the onion and lime juice. In a medium bowl, combine the orange sections with their juice, jicama, and cucumber.

2. With gloves, remove the stem from the pepper, slit it, and scrape out the seeds with a small sharp knife. Chop the flesh finely and add to the mandarin bowl. Alternatively, you can add the chili pepper.

3. Add the onion and lime juice to the mandarin bowl and mix well.

4. Cover and let stand at room temperature for at least 1 hour before serving.

NUTRITIONAL IMPACT PER SERVING: 1.4 g protein, 0.24 g fat, 18 g carbohydrates, 7 g fiber, 28 mg calcium, 288 mg potassium, 6 mg sodium, 0 mcg B12, 0.04 g leucine, 43 mg vitamin C, 75 calories

Hummus a Few Bars

(Gluten-free, dairy-free, vegetarian, vegan)

Serve this hummus with multicolored carrots, sliced cucumbers, other crudité, or papadams, high-protein bean-flour crackers.

8 SERVINGS

1 can (15 ounces) low-sodium chickpeas, drained and rinsed

1 teaspoon tahini or extra-virgin olive oil

1 cooked beet, diced (cook your own or buy beets ready to eat)

1 tablespoon freshly grated ginger

3 cloves garlic, finely minced (about 1 tablespoon)

2 tablespoons lemon juice

Salt to taste

Beet powder (optional)

1. In a food processor, combine all the ingredients and process until smooth.

2. You can add more pink color with beet powder.

NUTRITIONAL IMPACT PER SERVING: 3 g protein, 1 g fat, 8 g carbohydrates, 2 g fiber, 22 mg calcium, 96 mg potassium, 84 mg sodium, 0 mcg B12, 0.19 g leucine, 1 mg vitamin C, 54 calories

Tips and Secrets

Reserve the aquafaba liquid (that's the liquid that the chickpeas come packed in) to use as a vegan egg substitute. Three tablespoons of the liquid equals one egg.

Dressing and Sauces

Once you get the hang of preparing your own meals, you'll probably be inspired to experiment with new flavors to keep salads, vegetables, grains, and proteins interesting and enticing.

Sadly, most bottled sauces and even salad dressings are loaded with sugar. (Take a look at your favorite bottled salad dressing; you'll probably be dismayed to find "water" and "sugar" among the top three ingredients.) So, if you've already made the leap into healthy cooking, why not go a bit further by preparing your own?

Gilligan's Island Dressing and Marinade

(Gluten-free, dairy-free, vegetarian, vegan)

Perfect for when you're marooned on a tropical island with Ginger. This combines that spicy root with citrus fruits, adding punch to green salads, fruit salads, and cold pasta dishes; it can also serve as a marinade for chicken or fish.

8 SERVINGS (A LITTLE MORE THAN 2 TEASPOONS PER SERVING)

3 tablespoons orange juice
½ teaspoon ground ginger
¼ teaspoon orange zest
1 teaspoon ground cinnamon

¼ teaspoon ground nutmeg
3 tablespoons walnut, canola,
   or vegetable oil

1. In a bowl, use a hand blender to mix the orange juice, ginger, orange zest, cinnamon, and nutmeg.

2. Whisk in oil until blended.

NUTRITIONAL IMPACT PER SERVING: 0.07 g protein, 5 g fat, 1 g carbohydrates, 0.22 g fiber, 4 mg calcium, 15 mg potassium, 0.13 mg sodium, 0 mcg B12, 0 g leucine, 3 mg vitamin C, 49 calories

Truffles Right Here in River City
(Gluten-free, dairy-free, vegetarian, vegan)

The earthy taste of truffles smooths out the bite of high-quality olive oil. Use this dressing on a salad; over pasta, potatoes, or risotto; on sautéed mushrooms or other vegetables; or to finish off meat dishes for another level of flavor.

10 SERVINGS

2 tablespoons scallions, finely sliced

1 tablespoon white vinegar

1 tablespoon fresh lemon juice

1 teaspoon mustard powder

¼ cup extra-virgin olive oil

2 tablespoons truffle olive oil

Salt and white pepper to taste

1. Combine the scallions, vinegar, lemon juice, and mustard powder in a glass bowl.

2. In a separate bowl, combine the oils, then slowly add to the vinegar mix, whisking constantly to combine.

3. Add salt and white pepper to taste.

NUTRITIONAL IMPACT PER SERVING: 0.03 g protein, 8 g fat, 0.18 g carbohydrates, 0.04 g fiber, 1 mg calcium, 5 mg potassium, 0.57 mg sodium, 0 mcg B12, 0 g leucine, 0.46 mg vitamin C, 73 calories

Cherry Bomb Vinaigrette

(Gluten-free, dairy-free, vegetarian, vegan)

Use as a salad dressing or when cooking a flavorful fish like salmon.
Just put a few tablespoons on top before baking.

10 SERVINGS

5 fresh or frozen pitted sweet
  cherries
1 shallot, finely minced (½ cup)
1 tablespoon red wine

1 tablespoon balsamic vinegar
8 tablespoons extra-virgin
  olive oil
Salt and pepper to taste

1. With a food processor, mortar and pestle, or potato masher,
pulverize the cherries until pureed.

2. In a bowl, combine the shallots, wine, and vinegar and add the
cherry mixture. Whisk until combined.

3. Gradually add the olive oil while whisking continuously until
completely combined.

4. Add salt and pepper to taste.

NUTRITIONAL IMPACT PER SERVING: 0.23 g protein, 11 g fat,
2 g carbohydrates, 0.28 g fiber, 4 mg calcium, 39 mg potassium,
1 g sodium, 0 g B12, 0.01 g leucine, 0.85 vitamin C, 107 calories

Thyme in a Bottle

(Gluten-free, dairy-free, vegetarian, vegan)

Make a batch and keep on hand as this can be stored up to one week and used as a salad dressing, dip, or marinade for meat, chicken, or grilled veggies.

14 SERVINGS

¾ cup extra-virgin olive oil
2 tablespoons red wine vinegar
¼ cup white wine vinegar
1 tablespoon lemon juice
2 teaspoons fresh or bottled garlic, minced

¼ teaspoon crushed red pepper flakes
¼ teaspoon dried thyme
¼ teaspoon dried oregano
Kosher or sea salt and ground black pepper to taste

In a glass bowl, whisk together all the ingredients. Season with salt and pepper.

NUTRITIONAL IMPACT PER SERVING: 0.01 g protein, 12 g fat, 0.54 g carbohydrates, 0.03 g fiber, 1 mg calcium, 6 mg potassium, 0.72 mg sodium, 0 mcg B12, 0 g leucine, 0.25 mg vitamin C, 107 calories

Fun Fact

FRANKLY, I'D RATHER HAVE BULLETS: In the Middle Ages, sprigs of thyme—representing courage and bravery—were traditionally offered to soldiers going into battle.

Chimichurri in a Hurry

(Gluten-free, dairy-free, vegetarian, vegan)

Chimichurri sauce is commonly used in Latin American countries with BBQ meats and meat-and-vegetable skewers, but it can also be used as a condiment; a marinade for chicken, pork, or vegetables; a dressing for roasted potatoes; or as a spread on a toasted bread like bruschetta. Another novel use: as a very garlicky, spicy base for potato or pasta salad.

You can store this three to four days in the refrigerator.

8 SERVINGS

¾ cup extra-virgin olive oil

2 to 4 tablespoons red wine vinegar (to taste)

6 large cloves garlic, minced, or 2 heaping teaspoons bottled minced garlic or smoked garlic

¼ cup fresh parsley, chopped

¼ cup fresh cilantro, chopped (optional)

2 tablespoons fresh or dried oregano

1 teaspoon smoked paprika

Pinch crushed red pepper flakes

Salt to taste

1. In a food processor, grind all the ingredients until desired texture.

2. Adjust the seasoning and garlic to taste.

NUTRITIONAL IMPACT PER SERVING: 0.32 g protein, 20 g fat, 2 g carbohydrates, 1 g fiber, 20 mg calcium, 40 mg potassium, 3 mg sodium, 0 mcg B12, 0.02 g leucine, 3 mg vitamin C, 187 calories

Hey, Mamba!

(Gluten-free, dairy-free, vegetarian)

In Haiti, *mamba*—spicy peanut butter—is often used on veggie salads, grilled meats, tofu dishes, and even cold spring rolls. To make a thicker sauce, you can replace half the water with light coconut milk.

10 SERVINGS

½ cup peanut butter
2 cloves garlic
2 tablespoons lime juice
1 tablespoon honey

1 serrano chile (or use a milder pepper like jalapeño, if you prefer)
½ cup warm water
Salt to taste

1. In a blender, process all the ingredients until smooth.

2. Store until ready to use.

NUTRITIONAL IMPACT PER SERVING: 3 g protein, 7g fat, 5 g carbohydrates, 1 g fiber, 8 mg calcium, 80 mg potassium, 55 mg sodium, 0 mcg B12, 0 g leucine, 1 mg vitamin C, 85 calories

That's So Coulis

(Gluten-free, dairy-free, vegetarian, vegan)

Made from such simple ingredients, a red pepper coulis—a fancy word for vegetable or fruit puree—can add eye-popping, tongue-popping color and flavor to an otherwise more ordinary dish. You can use either orange or red peppers (green and yellow peppers are not as sweet) depending on the colors of the entire dish. Try putting the coulis in an icing bag or squeeze bottle to drizzle in a zig-zag pattern on soup, fish, or any food you are looking to take up a notch. Of course, you can just spoon it on as well.

6 SERVINGS

3 large red bell peppers, whole
2 tablespoons extra-virgin olive oil

1 shallot, finely sliced (½ cup)
1 tablespoon vinegar
Salt and white pepper to taste

1. Heat grill or preheat oven to 350°F.

2. Grill the peppers or roast them on a rimmed baking sheet for 20 minutes each side, until browned.

3. Take out the seeds and core and dice the peppers into ¼-inch pieces.

4. In a food processor, combine the peppers with the olive oil, shallot, and vinegar.

5. Push the mixture through a strainer into a bowl.

6. Season with salt and white pepper to taste.

NUTRITIONAL IMPACT PER SERVING: 1 g protein, 5 g fat, 7 g carbohydrates, 2 g fiber, 11 mg calcium, 219 mg potassium, 5 mg sodium, 0 mcg B12, 0.05 g leucine, 106 mg vitamin C, 75 calories

Fun Fact

LET'S GET ALONG: Oil and vinegar don't mix, unless you add a third ingredient such as mustard or egg yolk.

Sofrito, So Good

(Gluten-free, dairy-free, vegetarian, vegan)

This sauce is often used in Latin America and the Caribbean islands as a base for stews and soups and many other dishes, including those of chicken, pork, rice, or beans. It can be stored in the refrigerator for three to four days.

6 SERVINGS

2 tablespoons extra-virgin olive oil

1 cup white onion, chopped

1 cup mixed red, yellow, orange bell peppers, chopped

1½ cups cherry tomatoes, sliced

1 teaspoon smoked paprika

Salt to taste

5 cloves garlic, minced (or more to taste)

1½ cups fresh cilantro, chopped

1. In a large sauté pan, heat the olive oil over medium heat. Add the onions, peppers, tomatoes, paprika, and salt. Stir well and cook, uncovered, over low heat for 15 minutes.

2. Add the garlic and cook 5 more minutes, stirring often. Add the cilantro and mix into the rest of the sauce. Serve hot.

NUTRITIONAL IMPACT PER SERVING: 1 g protein, 5 g fat, 6 g carbohydrates, 2 g fiber, 15 mg calcium, 209 mg potassium, 6 mg sodium, 0 mcg B12, 0.03 g leucine, 40 mg vitamin C, 75 calories

Tips and Secrets

Make more than you need and then freeze in ice cube trays; you can then store the cubes in freezer bags and use as needed.

Snacks

Eating snacks that provide nutrients, protein, and fiber will help you feel satisfied until the next meal. Instead of eating mindlessly, eat purposefully. Plan on snacking with food that tastes good and is nourishing. Your snack goals are to add more protein and fiber into your day; these choices each deliver at least 2 grams of fiber for no more than 300 calories.

Most of us don't "cook" our snacks, but these recipes are too good and too healthy to hold back. You'll find a list of "toss 'em together" snack options in Chapter 3, Easy Snacks for Busy People on page 46. Adjust your snacking based on your needs, hunger, and activity.

Chocolate Nut Butter Energy Bites
(Dairy-free, vegetarian, vegan)

These are easy to make, easy to keep, and easy to eat! Recognize that these are not low-calorie. Just the opposite; they are somewhat dense. So, do pay attention to how many you eat. Perhaps pair with a glass of milk or a latte and use them to help you be prepared for that after-work workout—or to recover from a workout!

MAKES 12

1 cup peanut butter
5 tablespoons maple syrup
⅓ cup all-purpose flour

⅓ cup unsweetened cocoa powder

1. Line a baking sheet with parchment paper.

2. In a small bowl, mix all the ingredients together, adding flour as needed until firm enough to roll balls.

3. With a 2-tablespoon cookie scoop, scoop and drop dough onto parchment paper. Then place in freezer for 30 minutes until firm.

4. Remove from the freezer, roll into balls, and serve.

NUTRITIONAL IMPACT PER SERVING: 6 g protein, 11 g fat, 14 g carbohydrates, 2 g fiber, 22 mg calcium, 173 mg potassium, 92 mg sodium, 0 mcg B12, 0.03 g leucine, 0 mg vitamin C, 167 calories

Tips and Tricks

To prevent sticking when storing, roll the balls in unsweetened cocoa powder. (For each 1 teaspoon of cocoa powder add 4 calories and 1 gram of carbohydrates to the nutritional analysis above.) Store in the freezer to keep firm.

Beg-for-Egg Cupcakes
(Vegetarian)

A flavorful and protein-packed snack. Pair a few with a piece of fruit to up the fiber. You could also prepare these for breakfast or as an hors d'oeuvre.

MAKES 12

Canola oil cooking spray
All-purpose flour, for dusting
1 cup onion, finely diced
¼ cup yellow bell pepper, diced
¼ cup red bell pepper, diced
¼ cup orange bell pepper, diced
¼ cup green bell pepper, diced
2 teaspoons fresh minced garlic, or bottled minced garlic, or smoked garlic

2 cups fresh spinach, finely chopped into ⅛-inch slices
2 eggs
1 cup egg whites (from a package) or 8 egg whites
¼ cup shredded low-fat mozzarella or almond cheese

1. Preheat oven to 325°F.

2. Place the paper cupcake holders in a 12-muffin tin. Spray with cooking spray and dust with flour.

3. Spray a sauté pan with cooking spray and heat. Sauté the onions and peppers until slightly soft but not mushy, 2 to 5 minutes, stirring constantly with wooden spoon. Add the garlic and cook another 30 seconds. Add the spinach and cook until just wilted.

4. Put the vegetable mixture in a medium bowl and allow to cool.

5. Whisk together the eggs and egg whites. Add cheese to egg mixture and combine with vegetables.

6. Pour evenly into muffin cups.

(RECIPE CONTINUES ON NEXT PAGE)

7. Bake for 20 to 25 minutes until tops are slightly firm and slightly browned.

8. Remove from the oven and serve warm, or store in refrigerator for three to four days.

NUTRITIONAL IMPACT PER CUPCAKE: 4 g protein, 1 g fat, 3 g carbohydrates, 1 g fiber, 31 mg calcium, 121 mg potassium, 66 mg sodium, 0.13 mcg B12, 0.2 g leucine, 20 mg vitamin C, 42 calories

Smarter Food Popcorn

(Gluten-free, dairy-free, vegetarian, vegan)

2 SERVINGS

⅓ cup popcorn kernels

1 tablespoon extra-virgin olive oil

¼ teaspoon salt

1 tablespoon nutritional yeast (or to your taste)

1. Pop the kernels in an air popper.

2. Drizzle with the olive oil.

3. Sprinkle with the salt and nutritional yeast.

4. Toss, then taste and add more nutritional yeast, if desired.

NUTRITIONAL IMPACT PER SERVING: 9 g protein, 9 g fat, 37 g carbohydrates, 11 g fiber, 0 mg calcium, 120 mg potassium, 293 mg sodium, 9 mcg B12, 0 g leucine, 0 mg vitamin C, 229 calories

RECIPE VARIATIONS

Other spices to consider adding: a tiny bit of cayenne pepper, chili powder and cumin, everything bagel seasoning, oregano and basil, black pepper, and turmeric.

Yes, Honey–Roasted Chickpeas

(Gluten-free, dairy-free, vegetarian)

Want something crunchy and sweet? Try these homemade honey-roasted chickpeas. Prefer savory? Instead of cinnamon and honey, flavor with garlic, salt, chili powder, and soy sauce (and use sesame oil instead of olive oil). The options are endless, easy—and rich with protein.

Keep seasoning to one teaspoon to avoid overpowering the taste. You can also experiment with sprinkling your flavoring of choice on the chickpeas once they come out of the oven.

2 SERVINGS

1 can (15 ounces) chickpeas (drain, rinse, and let dry), or cook from soaked and dried peas

1 teaspoon extra-virgin olive oil
1 teaspoon ground cinnamon
1 tablespoon honey

1. Preheat oven to 300°F.

2. In a small bowl, combine the chickpeas, olive oil, and cinnamon and then spread onto a rimmed baking sheet.

3. Bake for about 1 hour, stirring occasionally. Chickpeas should be crunchy all the way through, not soft in the middle.

4. When the chickpeas are done, let cool, then drizzle with honey.

NUTRITIONAL IMPACT PER SERVING: 9 g protein, 5 g fat, 39 g carbohydrates, 9 g fiber, 68 mg calcium, 150 mg potassium, 270 mg sodium, 0 mcg B12, 0.64 g leucine, 0.23 mg vitamin C, 230 calories

Cottage Cheese Sundae
(Gluten-free, vegetarian)

You may think of cottage cheese as a breakfast food, but in fact, it's also a protein-packed snack. You can buy cottage cheese in individual sizes for easy grab-and-go, or buy in larger containers and portion as you wish. Jazz it up with this simple recipe.

1 SERVING

½ cup 2% cottage cheese   ¼ cup mixed nuts
1 cup fresh strawberries, sliced

Spoon the cottage cheese into a cup or bowl, then top with the strawberries and nuts.

NUTRITIONAL IMPACT PER SERVING: 16 g protein, 13 g fat, 20 g carbohydrates, 4 g fiber, 169 mg calcium, 474 mg potassium, 398 mg sodium, 0.53 mcg B12, 1.1 g leucine, 85 mg vitamin C, 245 calories

Appendix 1

The Complete Whole Body Reset Mix 'N' Match Meal Maker

Exact nutrients can vary, so check labels. Our source is the U.S. Department of Agriculture's Agricultural Research Service Food Data Central.

Protein

Aim for 25 to 30 grams of protein per meal (generally 25 for women, 30 for men), 7 grams per snack. Choose two to three servings of dairy a day and two to three servings of omega-3-rich foods a week (salmon, tuna, mackerel, sardines, walnuts, tofu).

DAIRY	SERVING SIZE	PROTEIN (GRAMS)
Cheese	1 oz	4–7
Cottage cheese	1 cup	22–25
Goat milk	8 oz	8
Kefir yogurt drink	1 cup	10
Milk (skim, 1%, 2%, whole)	1 cup	8
Ricotta cheese	¼ cup	5
Yogurt, flavored	1 cup	8
Yogurt, Greek, flavored	1 cup	19
Yogurt, Greek, plain	1 cup	22
Yogurt, plain	1 cup	9

PLANT-BASED PROTEIN	SERVING SIZE	PROTEIN (GRAMS)
Almond milk	1 cup	1
Beans, black (cooked or canned)	½ cup	8
Beans, pinto (cooked or canned)	½ cup	7
Black-eyed peas (cooked or canned)	½ cup	6
Chickpeas (garbanzo beans) (cooked or canned)	½ cup	7
Edamame (shelled)	½ cup	8
Hemp seeds	2 tbsp	7
Lentils, (cooked or canned)	½ cup	8
Nut butter (almond, peanut)	2 tbsp	6–8
Nuts	1 oz	4–7
Oat milk	1 cup	2
Pea-protein milk	1 cup	8
Pumpkin seeds	1 oz	8
Seitan	4 oz	28
Soy milk	1 cup	6
Tempeh	3 oz	16
Tofu, firm	6 oz (¾ cup)	16
Tofu, soft	6 oz (¾ cup)	15
Veggie burger	1 patty	10–15

SEAFOOD	SERVING SIZE	PROTEIN (GRAMS)
Anchovies (canned)	2 oz	13
Catfish	4 oz	15
Clams	3 oz	16
Crab	3 oz	15
Fish, smoked (herring, lox)	2 oz	10
Mackerel	3 oz	20

SEAFOOD	SERVING SIZE	PROTEIN (GRAMS)
Mussels	3 oz	20
Octopus	3 oz	13
Oysters	6	5
Salmon (canned)	3 oz	17
Salmon (cooked)	3 oz	23
Sardines	1 can (3¾ oz)	26
Scallops	3 oz	20
Shrimp/prawns	3 oz	12
Tuna, chunk light in water	3 oz	14
Whitefish	3 oz	14

MEAT	SERVING SIZE	PROTEIN (GRAMS)
Bacon, pork	2 slices	3
Bacon, turkey	2 slices	5
Beef, ground (85% lean)	4 oz	21
Beef jerky	1 oz	11
Bison (ground or steak)	4 oz	24
Chicken breast	3 oz	24
Duck	3 oz	17
Egg	1	6
Egg whites	2	7
Ham, deli sliced	3 oz	17
Ham, sliced	3 oz	12
Hot dog, beef	1	7
Lamb rack	4 oz	23
Pork loin and chop	3 oz	21
Sausage	3 oz	16

MEAT	SERVING SIZE	PROTEIN (GRAMS)
Steak (filet, porterhouse, sirloin, strip, T-bone)	4 oz	25
Turkey breast	3 oz	16
Turkey burger	3-oz patty	16
Turkey, deli sliced	3 slices	7
Veal cutlet, lean	3 oz	30
Venison	3 oz	31

HIGH-PROTEIN GRAINS (COOKED)	SERVING SIZE	PROTEIN (GRAMS)
Buckwheat groats (kasha)	1 cup	6
Pasta, chickpea	1 cup	14
Pasta, lentil	1 cup	11
Pasta, wheat	1 cup	8
Quinoa	1 cup	4
Soba noodles	1 cup	6
Wild rice	1 cup	6

Vegetables

Aim for 1½ to 2½ cups a day for fiber as well as protein; choose a variety of colors for different nutrients.

VEGETABLE	SERVING SIZE	PROTEIN (GRAMS)	FIBER (GRAMS)
Green			
Arugula	1 cup raw	1	0
Bok choy	1 cup raw	1	1
Broccoli	1 cup raw	3	2
Brussels sprouts	1 cup raw	3	3
Cabbage	1 cup raw	1	2
Collard greens	1 cup raw	1	1
Green beans	1 cup cooked	1	3
Kale	1 cup raw	1	1
Lettuce (bibb, butterhead, leaf, romaine)	1 cup raw	0	1
Mustard and turnip greens	1 cup raw	2	2
Spinach	1 cup raw	1	1
Swiss chard	1 cup raw	1	1
Red and Orange			
Beets	½ cup cooked	1	1
Carrots	1 medium or 7 baby carrots	1	2
Red, orange, yellow peppers	1 cup raw	1	3
Tomato	1 cup raw	2	2
Other			
Artichoke	1	3	7
Asparagus	5 medium spears	2	2
Bamboo shoots	1 cup raw	4	3
Bean sprouts	1 cup raw	3	2

VEGETABLE	SERVING SIZE	PROTEIN (GRAMS)	FIBER (GRAMS)
Cauliflower	1 cup raw	2	2
Celery	3 stalks/1 cup raw	1	2
Chile peppers	3	0	0
Corn (also a starch)	½ cup kernels	3	2
Cucumbers	1 cup raw	1	1
Eggplant	1 cup cooked	1	3
Fennel	½	2	4
Jicama	1 cup raw		6
Leeks	1 cup raw	1	2
Mushrooms	1 cup raw	2	1
Okra	1 cup cooked	3	5
Onion	½ each	1	1
Parsnips (also a starch)	1 cup raw	2	7
Peas (also a starch)	½ cup cooked	4	4
Radish	½ cup	0	1
Snap peas	½ cup raw	2	2
Snow peas	½ cup raw	2	2
Sunchoke	1 cup raw	3	2
Tomatillo	1 medium	0	1
Turnip	1	1	2
Water chestnuts (canned)	½ cup sliced	1	2
Winter squash (acorn, butternut) (also a starch)	1 cup raw	1	3
Zucchini, yellow squash	1 medium	2	2

Fruit

Aim for two to four servings a day.

FRUIT	SERVING SIZE	FIBER (GRAMS)
Apple	1 medium	5
Apricots	3	2
Asian pear	1	10
Banana	1 medium	3
Blackberries	1 cup	4
Blueberries	1 cup	4
Chayote	½ cup	1
Cherries	12	2
Coconut, dried	¼ cup	3
Cranberries, dried	22	1
Currants, dried	2 tbsp	1
Dates	3 small Deglet Noor or 1 large Medjool	2
Figs	2	3
Grapefruit	½	3
Grapes	17	1
Guava	1	3
Jackfruit	½ cup	2
Kiwi	2	4
Lemon	1	2
Lime	1	2
Lychee	10	1
Mango	½	2
Melon, cantaloupe, honeydew	1 cup	1
Nectarine	1	2
Orange	1	4
Papaya	1 cup	3

FRUIT	SERVING SIZE	FIBER (GRAMS)
Passion fruit	1	2
Peach	1	2
Pear	1	6
Persimmon	1	6
Pineapple	½ cup	1
Plantain	1	3
Plum	2	2
Pomegranate seeds	½ cup	3
Prunes	3	2
Raisins	1 small box (1½ oz)	2
Raspberries	1 cup	10
Star fruit	1 small	2
Strawberries	1 cup	3
Tamarind	1 oz	1
Tangerines	2	4
Watermelon	1¼ cups	1

Fiber-Rich Starches

Aim for four to eight servings a day.

FIBER-RICH STARCH	SERVING SIZE	FIBER (GRAMS)	PROTEIN (GRAMS)
Barley (cooked)	⅓ cup	2	1
Black beans (canned)	½ cup	9	8
Brown rice (cooked)	⅓ cup		2
Bulgur wheat (cooked)	½ cup	3	2
Cassava	½ cup raw	2	2
Cereal, breakfast (varies by brand—check package)	1 cup		
Chapati	1	5	4
Chickpea pasta	1 oz dry, ½ cup cooked	4	7
Corn	½ cup kernels	2	2
Corn tortilla	1	1	2–3
Crackers, multigrain (varies by brand—check package)			
Edamame, shelled	½ cup	4	8
English muffin, whole wheat	1	3	5
Grits, cooked	½ cup	1	2
Hominy, canned	¾ cup	3	2
Hummus	⅓ cup	5	5
Lima beans	½ cup	6	7
Naan bread, whole wheat	⅓ bread		0
Oatmeal, cooked	½ cup	2	2
Parsnips	1 cup raw	2	7
Peas	½ cup	4	4
Pita bread, whole wheat	1 small pita	2	3
Polenta (cooked)	½ cup	1	1
Popcorn	2½ cups air-popped	3	3

APPENDIX 1

FIBER-RICH STARCH	SERVING SIZE	FIBER (GRAMS)	PROTIEN (GRAMS)
Potato (sweet or white)	½ potato	2–3	1–2
Pumpkin (canned)	1 cup	7	3
Quinoa	½ cup cooked	2	4
Red lentil pasta	1 oz dry, ½ cup cooked	3–5	4–6
Whole wheat bread	1 slice	2–3	4–5
Whole wheat pasta	1 oz dry, ½ cup cooked	2	4
Whole wheat tortilla	1 medium	4	3
Winter squash (acorn, butternut)	1 cup raw	3	1

10-Day Reset Plan for Your Whole Body

BREAKFASTS

Waffle Topped with Cottage Cheese, Fruit, and Seeds

1 whole grain frozen waffle, ¾ cup 2% cottage cheese, 1 cup raspberries, 1 tbsp pumpkin seeds, 10 almonds

26 g protein, 10 g fiber, 398 calories

Wasa'p, New York? (recipe, page 238)

27 g protein, 10 g fiber, 427 calories

Yogurt Parfait

1 cup plain nonfat Greek yogurt, 1¼ cups frozen mixed berries (let thaw so juices seep into the yogurt), ¼ cup walnuts, 2 tbsp muesli

30 g protein, 9 g fiber, 442 calories

Scrambled Eggs with Potatoes and Fruit

2 large eggs scrambled with 1 oz part-skim mozzarella cheese, 1 cup roasted potatoes, ¼ cup chopped green pepper, and 1 tbsp onion in 2 tsp olive oil, served with 1 cup fruit (such as mango).

25 g protein, 5 g fiber, 535 calories

Avocado Toast with Yogurt and Blueberries

1 slice whole wheat toast with ⅓ cup mashed avocado, topped with your choice of spice mix (such as "everything bagel" mix)
1 cup plain nonfat Greek yogurt with 1 cup blueberries

29 g protein, 10 g fiber, 434 calories

Starbucks: Hearty Blueberry Oatmeal + Spinach, Feta & Cage-Free Egg White Breakfast Wrap

25 g protein, 8 g fiber, 510 calories

The Bogart Bowl (recipe, page 259)

25 g protein, 7 g fiber, 483 calories

Scramblin' Around Tofu (recipe, page 254)

Plus, 1 kiwi

31 g protein, 18 g fiber, 552 calories

Kale and Hearty Smoothie (recipe, page 244)

25 g protein, 7 g fiber, 374 calories

High-Protein Cereal and Nuts

¾ cup of cereal such as Kay's Naturals, Kashi Go Rise, or Special K Protein with 4 walnuts and ½ cup 1% milk, served with 4 oz vanilla Greek yogurt and 1 orange

27 g protein, 17 g fiber (approximate; varies by cereal brand), 437 calories

SNACKS

2 Beg-for-Egg Cupcakes (recipe, page 335)

Plus, 2 passion fruit

9 g protein, 6 g fiber, 119 calories

Legume-based Snack Chips (such as Biena Chickpea Puffs, The Good Bean Crunchy Chickpeas, or Bada Bean Bada Boom Crunchy Broad Beans) with 1 cup fruit

Nutritional data varies by brand

Protein Bar (such as Kind Protein Bar, Almond Butter Dark Chocolate; 88 Acres Banana Bread Protein Bar; or Go Macro Oatmeal Chocolate Chip)

Nutritional data varies by brand

Cottage Cheese with Berries and Nuts

½ cup 2% cottage cheese, 1 cup strawberries, ¼ cup mixed nuts
20 g protein, 5 g fiber, 353 calories

Trail Mix

2 tsp pumpkin seeds, 2 tbsp dried tart cherries, 13 almonds, ¼ cup whole wheat Chex-style cereal, 4 dried apricot halves
7 g protein, 6 g fiber, 282 calories

Yogurt and Nuts

1 cup vanilla Greek yogurt and 2 tbsp almonds
25 g protein, 3 g fiber, 294 calories

Open-faced Almond Butter Sandwich

1 tbsp almond butter on 1 slice whole wheat toast
With 8 oz sugar-free latte
14 g protein, 5 g fiber, 288 calories

Hummus a Few Bars (recipe, page 322)

With 1 cup sliced raw vegetables (such as carrots, cucumber, red peppers)
7 g protein, 8 g fiber, 158 calories

Blueberry Kefir (1 cup)

Plus, 1 apple

11 g protein, 4 g fiber, 235 calories

Smarter Food Popcorn (recipe, page 337)

9 g protein, 11 g fiber, 229 calories

LUNCHES

Cup of Lentil Soup (Canned or Homemade) with a Greek Salad

1½ cups romaine lettuce, ¼ cup cucumber, ¼ cup sliced onion, ⅛ cup green bell pepper, 2 oz feta cheese, 1 tbsp oil-and-vinegar dressing

25 g protein, 15 g fiber, 474 calories

Sushi, Sashimi, Edamame, and Seaweed Salad

1 tuna sushi maki roll, 1 salmon sashimi, 1 cup edamame, 1 seaweed salad

38 g protein, 7 g fiber, 371 calories

Panera Bread: Green Goddess Cobb Salad with Chicken

41 g protein, 8 g fiber, 530 calories

Cheese Sandwich with Side Salad and Pear

Sandwich: 2 slices whole grain bread, 2 slices Swiss cheese, 1 tsp mustard, 1 slice tomato
Salad: 1 cup mixed greens, ½ cup cucumber, 1½ tsp balsamic dressing
Plus, 1 pear

25 g protein, 14 g fiber, 552 calories

Turkey Sandwich with Carrot Sticks and Apple

Sandwich: 2 slices whole grain bread, 3 oz turkey, 1 tsp mayo
Plus, carrot sticks and 1 apple

26 g protein, 13 g fiber, 419 calories

Panda Express: Vegetable Spring Roll (appetizer) + Honey Walnut Shrimp + Super Greens

22 g protein, 9 g fiber, 640 calories

Quinoa Salad with Feta Cheese, Chickpeas, and Vegetables

¾ cup quinoa, ½ cup chickpeas, 1 oz pumpkin seeds, 1 oz feta cheese, ½ cup cucumber, ½ cup red bell pepper, ¼ cup chopped onion, 2 tsp lemon juice, 2 tsp olive oil

25 g protein, 12 g fiber, 622 calories

Subway: Turkey & Bacon Guacamole Sub

49 g protein, 9 g fiber, 511 calories

Grilled Chicken on Bed of Salad

4 oz chicken, 2 cups arugula, ¼ cup shaved fennel, ½ cup steamed broccoli, 3 tbsp pomegranate seeds, ½ cup black beans with 1 tbsp olive oil and 1 tsp lemon juice, salt and pepper to taste

31 g protein, 13 g fiber, 559 calories

Taco Bell: Power Menu Bowl with Chicken

26 g protein, 7 g fiber, 470 calories

DINNERS

A Chicken in Every Pot (recipe, page 297)

Plus, ½ cup pineapple

32 g protein, 18 g fiber, 483 calories

Shrimp and Pasta Primavera in Garlic Oil

Mix 3 oz cooked shrimp with 1 cup cooked penne pasta, ¼ cup steamed broccoli, ½ cup cooked spinach, ¼ cup steamed shredded carrots, and 2 tbsp Parmesan cheese and heat in 1 tbsp olive oil with a bit of chopped garlic.

25 g protein, 8 g fiber, 436 calories

Steak with Roasted Sweet Potato and Roasted Broccoli

6-oz tenderloin (⅛-inch trim), cooked as preferred

1 small sweet potato and 1 cup broccoli florets roasted in 2 tsp olive oil

49 g protein, 5 g fiber, 656 calories

Vegetarian Stir-fry Plus Fruit

1 cup bok choy, ½ cup red bell pepper, ½ cup snap peas, and 1 cup edamame cooked in 2 tsp peanut oil. Drizzle with a dash of sesame oil and 1 tsp sesame seeds to flavor. Serve over ½ cup brown rice. Add fruit on the side (such as a nectarine).

27 g protein, 17 g fiber, 586 calories

Muscled-Up Pesto Pasta with Basil Turkey Meatballs (recipes, pages 269 and 270)

28 g protein, 8 g fiber, 512 calories

Cracker Barrel Old Country Store: Lemon Grilled Rainbow Trout + Turnip Greens Bowl

67 g protein, 8 g fiber, 580 calories

German Steak and Potato Salad (recipe, page 285)

42 g protein, 8 g fiber, 512 calories

Chik-fil-A: Spicy Southwest Salad

33 g protein, 8 g fiber, 450 calories

Grilled Salmon and Farm Stand Salad with Roasted Garlic Dressing

Farm Stand Salad (recipe, page 317)

5 oz salmon: 31g protein, 0 g fiber, 292 calories
Total: 37 g protein, 8 g fiber, 520 calories

Popeyes: Catfish Filet (2 pcs) + Red Beans & Rice (reg.)

29 g protein, 7 g fiber, 707 calories

Acknowledgments

This book would not have been possible without the encouragement, support, and vision of the AARP leadership, especially CEO Jo Ann Jenkins and Executive Vice President and Chief Communications and Marketing Officer Martha Boudreau. A special thank-you to AARP Senior Vice President and Editorial Director Myrna Blyth for conceiving and driving this project forward, and to AARP Books Director Jodi Lipson, who played an integral role each step of the way. Thank you also to Michelle Harris and Stephanie Abramson, who quadruple-checked every fact in this book to ensure accuracy.

We are indebted to Simon & Schuster vice president and executive editor Priscilla Painton, for making this book a reality, and her team at Simon & Schuster, including Associate Editor Hana Park, Assistant Director of Publicity Elizabeth Herman, Steve Bedford, and production.

This project came to fruition under the guidance of Richard Pine, literary agent for *The Whole Body Reset* and *The South Beach Diet*. Many of AARP's talented editors and designers stepped up to help carry the load, especially Bob Love, Neil Wertheimer, Lesley Palmer, and Scott Davis. Special thanks to Laurette Davis for keeping the whole on, and to Jeff Csatari for stepping in when the going got tough. Chefs Lisa Dorfman, Judy Marshall, Jackie Newgent, and Daisy Pagani, and dieticians Carol Driesman, Tamar Kane, Alyssa Resnick, and Diana Ushay helped us pull together a delectable selection of recipes.

ACKNOWLEDGMENTS

The Whole Body Reset got off the ground thanks to the enormous efforts of Susan Reinhard and her AARP Healthy Living team, including Jennifer Peed, Chuck Rainville, Teresa Keenan, Sarah Burrell, and Lynda Flowers; Sarah Lenz Lock, executive director of the Global Council on Brain Health, convened by AARP; Leslie Nettleford in the Office of General Counsel; the amazing team who helped turn Café 58 and Seasons Culinary Services into the Whole Body Reset test kitchen, especially Chris Coombe and Kenneth Galang, with the help of Ana Lenis in Business Operations; Julia Rossi, Tracy Sacks, Nicolas Gouffray, and other folks at AARP Studios; AARP's National Office Fitness Center General Manager Carla Punch and her Optum team; Raj Mody and Sara Gallant on our Social team; and so many dedicated AARP employees who helped coordinate and promote our drive to build awareness within the organization, including, but hardly limited to, Jeffrey VanDam, Nina Halper, Lesley White, and Nakia McKenzie.

Notes

The notes that follow offer a partial list of scientific papers and other references that we have relied on and that you might find helpful if you want to learn more about some of the science behind this plan. If we cited every paper referenced or sources, the list would come to thousands of entries, but here's a start.

Chapter 1: The Age-Defying Magic of Protein Timing

1. Mohammad Siahpush, Melissa Tibbits, Raees A. Shaikh, Gopal K. Singh, et al., "Dieting Increases the Likelihood of Subsequent Obesity and BMI Gain: Results from a Prospective Study of an Australian National Sample," *International Journal of Behavioral Medicine* 22, no. 5 (October 2015): 662–71. https://pubmed.ncbi.nlm.nih.gov/25608460/.

2. Jamie I. Baum, Il-Young Kim, Robert R. Wolfe, "Protein Consumption and the Elderly: What Is the Optimal Level of Intake?" *Nutrients* 8, no. 6 (2016): 359, https://www.ncbi.nlm.nih.gov/pmc/articles/PMC4924200/; Rachel R. Deer and Elena Volpi, "Protein Intake and Muscle Function in Older Adults," *Current Opinion in Clinical Nutrition and Metabolic Care* 18, no. 3 (2015): 248–53. https://www.ncbi.nlm.nih.gov/pmc/articles/PMC4394186/; Julia Bollwein, Rebecca Diekmann, Matthias J. Kaiser, Jürgen M. Bauer, et al., "Distribution But Not Amount of Protein Intake Is Associated with Frailty: A Cross-Sectional Investigation in the Region of Nürnberg," *Nutrition Journal* 12 (August 5, 2013): 109. https://www.ncbi.nlm.nih.gov/pmc/articles/PMC3750269/.

3. Jinhee Kim, Yunhwan Lee, Seunghee Kye, Yoon-Sok Chung, et al., "Association of Vegetables and Fruits Consumption with Sarcopenia in Older Adults, the Fourth Korea National Health and Nutrition Examination Survey," *Age and Ageing* 44, no. 1 (January 2015). https://academic.oup.com/ageing/article/44/1/96/21279.

4. Paul J. Arciero, Rohan C. Edmonds, Kanokwan Bunsawat, Christopher L. Gentile, et al., "Protein-Pacing from Food or Supplementation Improves Physical Performance in Overweight Men and Women: The PRISE 2 Study," *Nutrients* 8,

no. 5 (2016): 288. https://www.ncbi.nlm.nih.gov/pmc/articles/PMC4882701/.

5. T. B. Symons, M. Sheffield-Moore, M. M. Mamerow, R. R. Wolfe, et al., "The Anabolic Response to Resistance Exercise and a Protein-Rich Meal Is Not Diminished by Age," *Journal of Nutrition, Health, and Aging* 15, no. 5 (May 2011): 376–81. https://pubmed.ncbi.nlm.nih.gov/21528164/.

6. Jürgen Bauer, Gianni Biolo, Tommy Cederholm, Matteo Cesari, et al., "Evidence-Based Recommendations for Optimal Dietary Protein Intake in Older People: A Position Paper from the PROT-AGE Study Group," *Journal of the American Medical Directors Association,* 14, no. 8 (August 2013): 542–49. https://www.sciencedirect.com/science/article/pii/S1525861013003265.

7. Interview with Jamie Baum, PhD, director of the Center for Human Nutrition at the University of Arkansas, Fayetteville.

8. Douglas Paddon-Jones and Blake B. Rasmussen, "Dietary Protein Recommendations and the Prevention of Sarcopenia," *Current Opinion in Clinical Nutrition and Metabolic Care* 12, no. 1 (January 2019): 86–90. https://pubmed.ncbi.nlm.nih.gov/19057193/.

9. Rosalba Putti, Raffaella Sica, Vincenzo Migliaccio, Lillà Lionetti, "Diet Impact on Mitochondrial Bioenergetics and Dynamics," *Frontiers in Physiology* 6 (April 8, 2015): 109. https://www.frontiersin.org/articles/10.3389/fphys.2015.00109/full.

Chapter 2: Our Changing Bodies, Our Changing Needs

1. A. M. Milan, R. F. D'Souza, S. Pundir, C. A. Pileggi, et al., "Older Adults Have Delayed Amino Acid Absorption after a High Protein Mixed Breakfast Meal," *Journal of Nutrition, Health, and Aging* 19, no. 8 (October 2015): 839–45. https://pubmed.ncbi.nlm.nih.gov/26412288/.

2. T. Brock Symons, Scott E. Schutzler, Tara L. Cocke, David L. Chinkes, et al. "Aging Does Not Impair the Anabolic Response to a Protein-Rich Meal," *American Journal of Clinical Nutrition* 86, no. 2 (August 2007): 451–56. https://doi.org/10.1093/ajcn/86.2.451.

3. Ian Janssen, "Influence of Sarcopenia on the Development of Physical Disability: The Cardiovascular Health Study," *Journal of the American Geriatrics Society* 54, no. 1 (January 2006): 56–62. https://pubmed.ncbi.nlm.nih.gov/16420198/.

4. W. Kyle Mitchell, John Williams, Philip Atherton, Mike Larvin, et al., "Sarcopenia, Dynapenia, and the Impact of Advancing Age on Human Skeletal Muscle Size and Strength; A Quantitative Review," *Frontiers in Physiology* 3 (2012): 260. https://www.ncbi.nlm.nih.gov/pmc/articles/PMC3429036/.

5. Matthew J. Delmonico, Tamara B. Harris, Marjolein Visser, Seok Won Park, et al., for the Health, Aging, and Body Composition Study, "Longitudinal Study of Muscle Strength, Quality, and Adipose Tissue Infiltration," *American Journal of Clinical Nutrition* 90, no. 6 (2009): 1579–85. https://www.ncbi.nlm.nih.gov/pmc/articles/PMC2777469/.

6. Stefanos Tyrovolas, Demosthenes Panagiotakos, Ekavi Georgousopoulou, Christina Chrysohoou, et al., "Skeletal Muscle Mass in Relation to 10 Year Cardiovascular Disease Incidence Among Middle Aged and Older Adults: The ATTICA Study," *Journal of Epidemiology and Community Health* 74, no. 1 (January 2020): 26–31. https://pubmed.ncbi.nlm.nih.gov/31712252/.

7. Ke-Vin Chang, Tsai-Hsuan Hsu, Wei-Ting Wu, Kuo-Chin Huang, et al., "Association Between Sarcopenia and Cognitive Impairment: A Systematic Review and Meta-Analysis," *Journal of the American Medical Directors Association* 17, no. 12 (December 1, 2016): 1164.e7–1164.e15. https://doi.org/10.1016/j.jamda.2016.09.013.

8. Ran Li, Jin Xia, X. I. Zhang, Wambui G. Gathirua-Mwangi, et al., "Associations of Muscle Mass and Strength with All-Cause Mortality Among US Older Adults," *Medicine and Science in Sports and Exercise* 50, no. 3 (March 2018): 458–67. https://www.ncbi.nlm.nih.gov/pmc/articles/PMC5820209/.

Chapter 3: Let's Spend a Day on the Whole Body Reset!

1. Eliana Zeballos and Jessica E. Todd, "The Effects of Skipping a Meal on Daily Energy Intake and Diet Quality," *Public Health Nutrition* 23, no. 18 (December 2020): 3346–55. https://pubmed.ncbi.nlm.nih.gov/32398192/.

2. Juliane Richter, Nina Herzog, Simon Janka, Thalke Baumann, et al., "Twice as High Diet-Induced Thermogenesis After Breakfast vs. Dinner on High-Calorie as Well as Low-Calorie Meals," *Journal of Clinical Endocrinology & Metabolism* 105, no. 3 (March 2020): dgz311. https://academic.oup.com/jcem/article/105/3/e211/5740411.

3. Daniela Jakubowicz, Maayan Barnea, Julio Wainstein, Oren Froy, "High Caloric Intake at Breakfast vs. Dinner Differentially Influences Weight Loss of Overweight and Obese Women," *Obesity* 21, no. 12 (December 2013): 2504–12. https://onlinelibrary.wiley.com/doi/full/10.1002/oby.20460.

Chapter 4: The Six Simple Secrets of Better Health

1. David S. Weigle, Patricia A. Breen, Colleen C. Matthys, Holly S. Callahan, et al., "A High-Protein Diet Induces Sustained Reductions in Appetite, Ad Libitum Caloric Intake, and Body Weight Despite Compensatory Changes in Diurnal Plasma Leptin and Ghrelin Concentrations," *American Journal of Clinical Nutrition* 82, no. 1 (July 2005): 41–48. https://academic.oup.com/ajcn/article/82/1/41/4863422; J. W. Apolzan, N. S. Carnell, R. D. Mattes, W. W. Campbell, "Inadequate Dietary Protein Increases Hunger and Desire to Eat in Younger and Older Men," *Journal of Nutrition* 137, no. 6 (2007): 1478–82. https://www.ncbi.nlm.nih.gov/pmc/articles/PMC2259459/.

2. Douglas Paddon-Jones, Eric Westman, Richard D. Mattes, Robert R. Wolfe, et al., "Protein, Weight Management, and Satiety," *American Journal of Clinical*

Nutrition 87, no. 5 (May 2008): 1558S–61S. https://academic.oup.com/ajcn/article/87/5/1558S/4650426.

3. S. Fujita and E. Volpi, "Amino Acids and Muscle Loss with Aging," *Journal of Nutrition* 136, no. 1 suppl. (2006): 277S–80S. https://www.ncbi.nlm.nih.gov/pmc/articles/PMC3183816/#R9; Douglas Paddon-Jones, Eric Westman, Richard D. Mattes, Robert R. Wolfe, et al., "Protein, Weight Management, and Satiety," *American Journal of Clinical Nutrition* 87, no. 5 (May 2008): 1558S–61S. https://doi.org/10.1093/ajcn/87.5.1558S.

4. T. B. Symons, M. Sheffield-Moore, R. R. Wolfe, D. Paddon-Jones, "A Moderate Serving of High-Quality Protein Maximally Stimulates Skeletal Muscle Protein Synthesis in Young and Elderly Subjects," *Journal American Diet Association* 109, no. 9 (September 2009): 1582–86. https://pubmed.ncbi.nlm.nih.gov/19699838/.

5. F. M. Martínez-Arnau, R. Fonfría-Vivas, O. Cauli, "Beneficial Effects of Leucine Supplementation on Criteria for Sarcopenia: A Systematic Review," *Nutrients* 11, no. 10 (2019): 2504. https://www.ncbi.nlm.nih.gov/pmc/articles/PMC6835605/.

6. Michaela C. Devries, Chris McGlory, Douglas R. Bolster, Alison Kamil, et al., "Leucine, Not Total Protein, Content of a Supplement Is the Primary Determinant of Muscle Protein Anabolic Responses in Healthy Older Women," *Journal of Nutrition* 148, no. 7 (July 2018): 1088–95. https://www.sciencedirect.com/science/article/pii/S1525861013003265, https://academic.oup.com/jn/article/148/7/1088/5036735.

7. A. J. Tessier and S. Chevalier, "An Update on Protein, Leucine, Omega-3 Fatty Acids, and Vitamin D in the Prevention and Treatment of Sarcopenia and Functional Decline," *Nutrients* 10, no. 8 (2018): 1099. https://www.ncbi.nlm.nih.gov/pmc/articles/PMC6116139/.

8. V. R. Young and P. L. Pellett, "Plant Proteins in Relation to Human Protein and Amino Acid Nutrition," *American Journal of Clinical Nutrition* 59, no. 5 suppl. (May 1994): 1203S–12S. https://academic.oup.com/ajcn/article-abstract/59/5/1203S/4732587?.

9. Meghan Meehan and Sue Penckofer, "The Role of Vitamin D in the Aging Adult," *Journal of Aging & Gerontology* 2, no. 2 (December 2014): 60–71. https://www.ncbi.nlm.nih.gov/pmc/articles/PMC4399494/.

10. Simone Radavelli-Bagatini, Kun Zhu, Joshua R Lewis, Satvinder S. Dhaliwal, et al., "Association of Dairy Intake with Body Composition and Physical Function in Older Community-Dwelling Women," *Journal of the Academy of Nutrition and Dietetics* 113, no. 12 (December 2013): 1669–74. https://www.ncbi.nlm.nih.gov/pubmed/23911336.

11. Mi-Hyun Kim, So Young Bu, Mi Kyeong Choi, "Daily Calcium Intake and Its Relation to Blood Pressure, Blood Lipids, and Oxidative Stress Biomarkers in Hypertensive and Normotensive Subjects," *Nutrition Research and*

Practice 6, no. 5 (2012): 421–28. https://www.ncbi.nlm.nih.gov/pmc/articles/PMC3506873/.

12. Kevin Li, Xia-Fang Wang, Ding-YouLi, Yuan-Cheng Chen, et al., "The Good, the Bad, and the Ugly of Calcium Supplementation: A Review of Calcium Intake on Human Health," *Clinical Interventions in Aging* 13 (2018): 2443–52. https://www.ncbi.nlm.nih.gov/pmc/articles/PMC6276611/.

13. S. M. Robinson, J. Y. Reginster, R. Rizzoli, S. C. Shaw, et al., "Does Nutrition Play a Role in the Prevention and Management of Sarcopenia?" *Clinical Nutrition* 37, no. 4 (2018): 1121–32. https://www.ncbi.nlm.nih.gov/pmc/articles/PMC5796643/; Marjolein Visser, Dorly J. H. Deeg, and Paul Lips, "Longitudinal Aging Study Amsterdam. Low Vitamin D and High Parathyroid Hormone Levels as Determinants of Loss of Muscle Strength and Muscle Mass (Sarcopenia): the Longitudinal Aging Study Amsterdam," *Journal of Clinical Endocrinology and Metabolism* 88, no. 12 (December 2003): 5766–72. https://www.ncbi.nlm.nih.gov/pubmed/14671166.

14. E. H. Reynolds, "Folic Acid, Ageing, Depression, and Dementia," *BMJ* 324, no. 7352 (June 22, 2002): 1512–15. https://www.ncbi.nlm.nih.gov/pmc/articles/PMC1123448/.

15. Yu Jiang, Sheng-Hui Wu, Xiao-Ou Shu, Yong-Bing Xiang, et al., "Cruciferous Vegetable Intake Is Inversely Correlated with Circulating Levels of Proinflammatory Markers in Women," *Journal of the Academy of Nutrition and Dietetics* 114, no. 5 (May 2014): 700–8.e2. https://www.ncbi.nlm.nih.gov/pmc/articles/PMC4063312/.

16. Fengmui Zhu, Bin Du, and Baojun Xu, "Anti-Inflammatory Effects of Phytochemicals from Fruits, Vegetables, and Food Legumes: A Review," *Critical Reviews in Food Science and Nutrition* 58, no. 8 (May 24, 2018): 1260–70. https://pubmed.ncbi.nlm.nih.gov/28605204/.

17. Sebastiaan Dalle, Lenka Rossmeislova, and Katrien Koppo, "The Role of Inflammation in Age-Related Sarcopenia," *Frontiers in Physiology* 8 (December 12, 2017): 1045. https://www.ncbi.nlm.nih.gov/pmc/articles/PMC5733049/.

18. Charlotte E. Neville, Ian S. Young, Sarah E. C. M. Gilchrist, Michelle C. McKinley, et al., "Effect of Increased Fruit and Vegetable Consumption on Physical Function and Muscle Strength in Older Adults," *Age (Dordr)* 35, no. 6 (2013): 2409–22. https://www.ncbi.nlm.nih.gov/pmc/articles/PMC3825010/.

19. Larry A. Tucker and Kathryn S. Thomas, "Increasing Total Fiber Intake Reduces Risk of Weight and Fat Gains in Women," *Journal of Nutrition* 139, no. 3 (March 2009): 576–81. https://academic.oup.com/jn/article/139/3/576/4670386.

20. Kristen G. Hairston, Mara Z. Vitolins, Jill M. Morris, Andrea M. Anderson, et al., "Lifestyle Factors and 5-Year Abdominal Fat Accumulation in a Minority Cohort: The IRAS Family Study," *Obesity* 20, no. 2 (February 2012): 421–27. https://onlinelibrary.wiley.com/doi/full/10.1038/oby.2011.171.

21. Chris McGlory, Philip C. Calder, and Everson A. Nunes, "The Influence of Omega-3 Fatty Acids on Skeletal Muscle Protein Turnover in Health, Disuse, and Disease," *Frontiers in Nutrition* 6, no. 144 (September 6, 2019): 144. https://www.ncbi.nlm.nih.gov/pmc/articles/PMC6742725/; Shichun Du, Jie Jin, Wenjun Fang, and Qing Su, "Does Fish Oil Have an Anti-Obesity Effect in Overweight/Obese Adults? A Meta-Analysis of Randomized Controlled Trials," *PLoS One* 10, no. 11 (2015):e0142652. https://www.ncbi.nlm.nih.gov/pmc/articles/PMC4646500/.

22. Azin Mohebi-Nejad and Behnood Bikdeli, "Omega-3 Supplements and Cardio-vascular Diseases," *Tanaffos* 13, no. 1 (2014): 6–14. https://www.ncbi.nlm.nih.gov/pmc/articles/PMC4153275/.

23. Giacomo Monzio Compagnoni, Alessio Di Fonzo, Stefania Corti, Giacomo P. Comi, et al., "The Role of Mitochondria in Neurodegenerative Diseases: The Lesson from Alzheimer's Disease and Parkinson's Disease," *Molecular Neurobiology* 57, no. 7 (July 2020): 2959–80. https://pubmed.ncbi.nlm.nih.gov/32445085/.

24. Simon N. Thornton, "Increased Hydration Can Be Associated with Weight Loss," *Frontiers in Nutrition* 3, no. 18 (June 10, 2016). https://www.ncbi.nlm.nih.gov/pmc/articles/PMC4901052/.

25. Marcus D. Goncalves, Changyuan Lu, Jordan Tutnauer, Travis E. Hartman, et al., "High-Fructose Corn Syrup Enhances Intestinal Tumor Growth in Mice," *Science* 22, no. 363 (March 22, 2019): 1345–49. https://science.sciencemag.org/content/363/6433/1345.

26. Francisco Javier Ruiz-Ojeda, Julio Plaza-Díaz, Maria Jose Sáez-Lara, and Angel Gil, "Effects of Sweeteners on the Gut Microbiota: A Review of Experimental Studies and Clinical Trials," *Advances in Nutrition* 10, suppl.1 (January 1, 2019): S31–S48. [Published correction appears in *Advances in Nutrition* 11, no. 2 (March 1, 2020): 468.]

27. Elizabeth Dennis, Ana Laura Dengo, Dana L. Comber, Kyle D. Flack, et al., "Water Consumption Increases Weight Loss During a Hypocaloric Diet Intervention in Middle-Aged and Older Adults," *Obesity* (Silver Spring) 18, no. 2 (February 2010): 300–7. https://pubmed.ncbi.nlm.nih.gov/19661958/.

Chapter 5: The Inside Story of Your Gut

1. Sebastiaan Dalle, Lenka Rossmeislova, and Katrien Koppo, "The Role of In-flammation in Age-Related Sarcopenia," *Frontiers in Physiology* 8 (December 12, 2017): 1045. https://www.ncbi.nlm.nih.gov/pmc/articles/PMC5733049/.

2. Priya Londhe and Denis C. Guttridge, "Inflammation Induced Loss of Skeletal Muscle," *Bone* 80 (2015): 131–42. https://www.ncbi.nlm.nih.gov/pmc/articles/PMC4600538/.

3. R. A. Whitmer, D. R. Gustafson, E. Barrett-Connor, M. N. Haan, et al., "Central Obesity and Increased Risk of Dementia More Than Three Decades Later," *Neurology* 71, no. 14 (September 30, 2008): 1057–64. https://pubmed.ncbi.nlm.nih.gov/18367704/.

4. Kira Leishear, Robert M. Boudreau, Stephanie A. Studenski, Luigi Ferrucci, et al., "The Relationship of Vitamin B12 and Sensory and Motor Peripheral Nerve Function in Older Adults," *Journal of the American Geriatrics Society* 60, no. 6 (2012): 1057–63. https://www.ncbi.nlm.nih.gov/pmc/articles/PMC3376015/.

5. Ravinder Nagpal, Rabina Mainali, Shokouh Ahmadi, Shaohua Wang, et al., "Gut Microbiome and Aging: Physiological and Mechanistic Insights," *Nutrition and Healthy Aging* 4, no. 4 (June 15, 2018): 267–85. https://www.ncbi.nlm.nih.gov/pmc/articles/PMC6004897/.

6. R. T. Liu, "The Microbiome as a Novel Paradigm in Studying Stress and Mental Health," *American Psychologist* 72, no. 7 (2017): 655–67. https://www.ncbi.nlm.nih.gov/pmc/articles/PMC5637404/.

7. Sara C. Di Rienzi and Robert A. Britton, "Adaptation of the Gut Microbiota to Modern Dietary Sugars and Sweeteners," *Advances in Nutrition* 11, no. 3 (May 2020): 616–29. https://academic.oup.com/advances/article/11/3/616/5614218.

8. Rosa Krajmalnik-Brown, Zehra-Esra Ilhan, Dae-Wook Kang, and John K. DiBaise, "Effects of Gut Microbes on Nutrient Absorption and Energy Regulation," *Nutrition in Clinical Practice* 27, no. 2 (2012): 201–14. https://www.ncbi.nlm.nih.gov/pmc/articles/PMC3601187/.

9. S. Boyd Eaton, "The Ancestral Human Diet: What Was It and Should It Be a Paradigm for Contemporary Nutrition?" *Proceedings of the Nutrition Society* 65, no. 1 (February 2006): 1–6. https://pubmed.ncbi.nlm.nih.gov/16441938/.

Chapter 6: How the Whole Body Reset Can Help Fight Disease and Save Your Life (Over and Over Again)

1. Global BMI Mortality Collaboration, Emanuele Di Angelantonio, Shilpa Bhupathiraju, David Wormser, et al., "Body-Mass Index and All-Cause Mortality: Individual-Participant-Data Meta-Analysis of 239 Prospective Studies in Four Continents," *Lancet* 388, no. 10046 (August 20, 2016): 776–86. https://pubmed.ncbi.nlm.nih.gov/27423262/.

2. Hanfei Xu, L. Adrienne Cupples, Andrew Stokes, and Ching-Ti Liu, "Association of Obesity with Mortality Over 24 Years of Weight History: Findings from the Framingham Heart Study," *JAMA Network Open* 1, no. 7 (2018): e184587.

3. Sina Naghshi, Omid Sadeghi, Walter C. Willett, and Ahmad Esmaillzadeh, "Dietary Intake of Total, Animal, and Plant Proteins and Risk of All Cause, Cardiovascular, and Cancer Mortality: Systematic Review and Dose-Response Meta-Analysis of Prospective Cohort Studies," *BMJ* 370 (July 22, 2020): m2412. https://www.bmj.com/content/370/bmj.m2412.

4. Philip C. Calder, Nabil Bosco, Raphaëlle Bourdet-Sicard, Lucile Capuron, et al., "Health Relevance of the Modification of Low Grade Inflammation in Ageing (Inflammageing) and the Role of Nutrition," *Ageing Research Reviews* 40 (November 2017): 95–119. https://www.sciencedirect.com/science/article/pii/S156816371730003X.

5. A. E. Buyken, V. Flood, M. Empson, E. Rochtchina, et al., "Carbohydrate Nutrition and Inflammatory Disease Mortality in Older Adults," *American Journal of Clinical Nutrition* 92, no. 3 (September 2010): 634–43. https://pubmed.ncbi .nlm.nih.gov/20573797/.

6. John A. Batsis, Todd A. Mackenzie, Jonathan D. Jones, Francisco Lopez-Jimenze, et al., "Sarcopenia, Sarcopenic Obesity and Inflammation: Results from the 1999–2004 National Health and Nutrition Examination Survey," *Clinical Nutrition* 35, no. 6 (December 2016): 1472–83. https://pubmed.ncbi.nlm.nih.gov/27091774/.

7. Niharika A. Duggal, Grace Niemiro, Stephen D. Richard Harridge et al., "Can Physical Activity Ameliorate Immunosenescence and Thereby Reduce Age-Related Multi-Morbidity?" *Nature Reviews Immunology* 19 (2019): 563–72. https://www.nature.com/articles/s41577-019-0177-9.

8. Hansongyi Lee, In Seok Lee, and Ryowon Choue, "Obesity, Inflammation and Diet," *Pediatric Gastroenterology, Hepatology & Nutrition* 16, no. 3 (2013): 143–52. https://www.ncbi.nlm.nih.gov/pmc/articles/PMC3819692/; A. Shuster, M. Patlas, J. H. Pinthus, and M. Mourtzakis, "The Clinical Importance of Visceral Adiposity: A Critical Review of Methods for Visceral Adipose Tissue Analysis," *British Journal of Radiology* 85, no. 1009 (January 2012): 1–10. https://www .ncbi.nlm.nih.gov/pmc/articles/PMC3473928/.

9. Hannah D. Holscher, "Dietary Fiber and Prebiotics and the Gastrointestinal Microbiota, *Gut Microbes* 8, no. 2 (2017): 172–84. https://www.ncbi.nlm.nih .gov/pmc/articles/PMC5390821/; D. Zheng, T. Liwinski, and E. Elinav, "Interaction Between Microbiota and Immunity in Health and Disease," *Cell Research* 30 (2020): 492–506. https://www.nature.com/articles/s41422-020-0332-7.

10. Alex Buoite Stella, Gianluca Gortan Cappellari, Rocco Barazzoni, and Michela Zanetti, "Update on the Impact of Omega-3 Fatty Acids on Inflammation, Insulin Resistance and Sarcopenia: A Review," *International Journal of Molecular Sciences* 19, no. 1 (January 11, 2018): 218. https://www.ncbi.nlm.nih.gov/pmc/ articles/PMC5796167/.

11. Karin Ried, Thomas Sullivan, Peter Fakler, Oliver R. Frank, et al., "Does Chocolate Reduce Blood Pressure? A Meta-Analysis," *BMC Medicine* 8, 39 (2010). https://bmcmedicine.biomedcentral.com/articles/10.1186/1741-7015-8-39.

12. G. C. Chen, D. B. Lv, Z. Pang, J-Y Dong, et al., "Dietary Fiber Intake and Stroke Risk: A Meta-Analysis of Prospective Cohort Studies," *European Journal of Clinical Nutrition* 67 (2013): 96–100. https://www.nature.com/articles/ ejcn2012158.

13. Enrique G. Artero, Duck-chul Lee, Carl J. Lavie, Vanesa España-Romero, et al., "Effects of Muscular Strength on Cardiovascular Risk Factors and Prognosis," *Journal of Cardiopulmonary Rehabilitation and Prevention* 32, no. 6 (2012): 351–58. https://www.ncbi.nlm.nih.gov/pmc/articles/PMC3496010/#R27.

14. A. L. Maslow, X. Sui, N. Colabianchi, J. Hussey, et al., "Muscular Strength and Incident Hypertension in Normotensive and Prehypertensive Men," *Medi-*

cine & Science in Sports & Exercise 42, no. 2 (February 2010): 288–95. https://pubmed.ncbi.nlm.nih.gov/19927030/.

15. Aurélie Ballon, Manuela Neuenschwander, and Sabrina Schlesinger, "Breakfast Skipping Is Associated with Increased Risk of Type 2 Diabetes among Adults: A Systematic Review and Meta-Analysis of Prospective Cohort Studies," *Journal of Nutrition* 149, no. 1 (January 2019): 106–13. https://academic.oup.com/jn/article/149/1/106/5167902.

16. Young-Min Park, Timothy D. Heden, Ying Liu, Lauryn M. Nyhoff, et al., "A High-Protein Breakfast Induces Greater Insulin and Glucose-Dependent Insulinotropic Peptide Responses to a Subsequent Lunch Meal in Individuals with Type 2 Diabetes," *Journal of Nutrition* 145, no. 3 (March 2015): 452–58. https://pubmed.ncbi.nlm.nih.gov/25733459/.

17. Preethi Srikanthan and Arun S. Karlamangla, "Relative Muscle Mass Is Inversely Associated with Insulin Resistance and Prediabetes. Findings from the Third National Health and Nutrition Examination Survey," *Journal of Clinical Endocrinology & Metabolism* 96, no. 9 (September 1, 2011): 2898–2903. https://academic.oup.com/jcem/article/96/9/2898/2834715.

18. Sotirios Tsalamandris, Alexios S. Antonopoulos, Evangelos Oikonomou, George-Aggelos Papamikroulis, et al., "The Role of Inflammation in Diabetes: Current Concepts and Future Perspectives," *European Cardiology Review* 14, no. 1 (2019): 50–59. https://www.ncbi.nlm.nih.gov/pmc/articles/PMC6523054/.

Chapter 7: How the Whole Body Reset Can Help Keep Your Mind Sharp

1. Matthew P. Pase, Jayandra J. Himali, Paul F. Jacques, Charles DeCarli, et al., "Sugary Beverage Intake and Preclinical Alzheimer's Disease in the Community," *Alzheimer's & Dementia* 13, no. 9 (September 2017): 955–64. https://alz-journals.onlinelibrary.wiley.com/share/YKFGBB5IW6HTNQR5KR6W?target=10.1016/j.jalz.2017.01.024.

2. Rachel K. Johnson, Lawrence J. Appel, Michael Brands, Barbara V. Howard, et al., "Dietary Sugars Intake and Cardiovascular Health: A Scientific Statement from the American Heart Association," *Circulation* 120 (2009): 1011–20. https://www.ahajournals.org/doi/pdf/10.1161/circulationaha.109.192627.

3. Karen W. Della Corte, Ines Perrar, Katharina J. Penczynski, Lukas Schwingshackl, et al., "Effect of Dietary Sugar Intake on Biomarkers of Subclinical Inflammation: A Systematic Review and Meta-Analysis of Intervention Studies," *Nutrients* 10, no. 5 (May 12, 2018): 606. https://www.ncbi.nlm.nih.gov/pmc/articles/PMC5986486/.

4. J. Li, D. H. Lee, J. Hu, F. K. Tabung, et al., "Dietary Inflammatory Potential and Risk of Cardiovascular Disease Among Men and Women in the U.S.," *Journal of the American College of Cardiology* 76, no. 19 (November 2020): 2181–93. https://pubmed.ncbi.nlm.nih.gov/33153576/.

5. Patricia A. Boyle, Aron S. Buchman, Robert S. Wilson, Sue E. Leurgans, et al., "Association of Muscle Strength with the Risk of Alzheimer's Disease and the Rate of Cognitive Decline in Community-Dwelling Older Persons," *Archives of Neurology* 66, no. 11 (2009): 1339–44. https://www.ncbi.nlm.nih.gov/pmc/articles/PMC2838435/.

6. Jahae Kim, Kang-Ho Choi, Sang-Geon Cho, Sae-Ryung Kang, et al., "Association of Muscle and Visceral Adipose Tissues with the Probability of Alzheimer's Disease in Healthy Subjects," *Scientific Reports* 9, no. 1 (January 30, 2019): 949. https://www.ncbi.nlm.nih.gov/pmc/articles/PMC6353958/.

Chapter 8: Your Magic Supermarket Label Decoder

1. Mahshid Dehghan, Andrew Mente, Sumathy Rangarajan, Patrick Sheridan, et al., "Association of Dairy Intake With Cardiovascular Disease and Mortality in 21 Countries from Five Continents (PURE): A Prospective Cohort Study," *Lancet* 392, no. 1016 (November 24, 2018): 2288–97. https://www.thelancet.com/journals/lancet/article/PIIS0140-6736(18)31812-9/fulltext.

Chapter 10: Toss Out Your Old Diet Books

1. Larry A. Tucker, "Dietary Fiber and Telomere Length in 5674 U.S. Adults: An NHANES Study of Biological Aging," *Nutrients* 10, no. 4 (April 2018): 400. https://www.ncbi.nlm.nih.gov/pmc/articles/PMC5946185/; Huda Adwan Shekhidem, Lital Sharvit, Eva Leman, Irena Manov, et al., "Telomeres and Longevity: A Cause or an Effect?", *International Journal of Molecular Sciences* 20, no. 13 (July 1, 2019): 3233. https://www.ncbi.nlm.nih.gov/pmc/articles/PMC6651551/.

2. Iolanda Cioffi, Andrea Evangelista, Valentina Ponzo, Giovannino Ciccone, et al., "Intermittent Versus Continuous Energy Restriction on Weight Loss and Cardiometabolic Outcomes: A Systematic Review and Meta-Analysis of Randomized Controlled Trials," *Journal of Translational Medicine* 16, no. 1 (December 24, 2018): 371. https://pubmed.ncbi.nlm.nih.gov/30583725/.

3. John F. Trepanowski, Cynthia M. Kroeger, Adrienne Barnosky, Monica C. Klempel, et al., "Effect of Alternate-Day Fasting on Weight Loss, Weight Maintenance, and Cardioprotection Among Metabolically Healthy Obese Adults: A Randomized Clinical Trial," *JAMA Internal Medicine* 177, no. 7 (2017): 930–38. https://jamanetwork.com/journals/jamainternalmedicine/fullarticle/2623528?utm_campaign=articlePDF&utm_medium=articlePDFlink&utm_source=articlePDF&utm_content=jamainternmed.2017.0936.

4. Dylan A. Lowe, Nancy Wu, Linnea Rohdin-Bibby, A. Holliston Moore, et al., "Effects of Time-Restricted Eating on Weight Loss and Other Metabolic Parameters in Women and Men With Overweight and Obesity: The TREAT Randomized Clinical Trial," *JAMA Internal Medicine* 180, no. 11 (November 1, 2020):1491–99. https://pubmed.ncbi.nlm.nih.gov/32986097/.

5. Pamela M. Peeke, Frank L. Greenway, Sonja K. Billes, Dachuan Zhang, et al., "Effect of Time Restricted Eating on Body Weight and Fasting Glucose in Participants with Obesity: Results of a Randomized, Controlled, Virtual Clinical Trial," *Nutrition and Diabetes* 11, no. 1 (January 15, 2021): 6. https://www.ncbi.nlm.nih.gov/pmc/articles/PMC7809455/.

6. Kevin D. Hall and Scott Kahan, "Maintenance of Lost Weight and Long-Term Management of Obesity," *Medical Clinics of North America* 102, no. 1 (2018): 183–97. https://www.ncbi.nlm.nih.gov/pmc/articles/PMC5764193/.

Chapter 11: The Metabolism Myth

1. Paddy C. Dempsey, Robyn N. Larsen, David W. Dunstan, Neville Owen, et al., "Sitting Less and Moving More: Implications for Hypertension," *Hypertension* 72, no. 5 (November 2018): 1037–46. https://www.ahajournals.org/doi/10.1161/HYPERTENSIONAHA.118.11190, https://www.researchgate.net/publication/328734018_Sitting_Less_and_Moving_More_Implications_for_Hypertension.

2. Martin Lövdén, Weili Xu, and Hui-Xin Wang, "Lifestyle Change and the Prevention of Cognitive Decline and Dementia: What Is the Evidence?" *Current Opinion in Psychiatry* 26, no. 3 (May 2013): 239–43. https://pubmed.ncbi.nlm.nih.gov/23493129/.

3. Vincenzo Monda, Ines Villano, Antonietta Messina, Anna Valenzano, et al., "Exercise Modifies the Gut Microbiota with Positive Health Effects," *Oxidative Medicine and Cellular Longevity* (2017): 3831972. https://www.ncbi.nlm.nih.gov/pmc/articles/PMC5357536/.

Chapter 12: Your Whole Body Fitness Plan

1. Seol-Jung Kang, Eon-ho Kim, and Kwang-Jun Ko, "Effects of Aerobic Exercise on the Resting Heart Rate, Physical Fitness, and Arterial Stiffness of Female Patients with Metabolic Syndrome," *Journal of Physical Therapy Science* 28, no. 6 (2016): 1764–68. https://www.ncbi.nlm.nih.gov/pmc/articles/PMC4932052/.

2. Jonathan Myers, "Exercise and Cardiovascular Health," *Circulation* 107, no. 1 (January 7, 2003): e2–e5. https://www.ahajournals.org/doi/pdf/10.1161/01.CIR.0000048890.59383.8D.

3. Mark T. Windsor, Tom G. Bailey, Maria Perissiou, Lara Meital, et al., "Cytokine Responses to Acute Exercise in Healthy Older Adults: The Effect of Cardiorespiratory Fitness," *Frontiers in Physiology* 9 (March 15, 2018): 203. https://www.frontiersin.org/articles/10.3389/fphys.2018.00203/full.

4. Liza Stathokostas, Matthew W. McDonald, Robert M. D. Little, and Donald H. Paterson, "Flexibility of Older Adults Aged 55–86 Years and the Influence of Physical Activity," *Journal of Aging Research* (2013): 743843. https://www.ncbi.nlm.nih.gov/pmc/articles/PMC3703899/.

Chapter 13: Troubleshooting the Whole Body Reset

1. Kevin D. Hall, Alexis Ayuketah, Robert Brychta, Hongyi Cai, et al., "Ultra-Processed Diets Cause Excess Calorie Intake and Weight Gain: An Inpatient Randomized Controlled Trial of Ad Libitum Food Intake," *Cell Metabolism* 30, no. 1 (July 2, 2019): 67–77. https://pubmed.ncbi.nlm.nih.gov/31105044/.

Chapter 14: Whole Body Recipes

1. Amy Banaszek, Jeremy R. Townsend, David Bender, William C. Vantrease, et al., "The Effects of Whey vs. Pea Protein on Physical Adaptations Following 8 Weeks of High-Intensity Functional Training (HIFT): A Pilot Study," *Sports (Basel)* 7, no. 1 (2019): 12. https://www.ncbi.nlm.nih.gov/pmc/articles/PMC6358922/.
2. Alec Coppen and Christina Bolander-Gouaille, "Treatment of Depression: Time to Consider Folic Acid and Vitamin B12," *Journal of Psychopharmacology* 19, no. 1 (January 2005): 59–65. https://pubmed.ncbi.nlm.nih.gov/15671130/.

List of Recipes

Breakfast

Cooked Breakfasts

Lunch and Dinner Entrees

Soups, Salads, and Sides

LIST OF RECIPES

Dressing and Sauces

Snacks

Index

About the Authors and AARP

Stephen Perrine is an executive editor of *AARP the Magazine* and the *AARP Bulletin*, where he oversees health, nutrition, and fitness coverage. He has worked on more than two dozen *New York Times* bestsellers in the diet and nutrition field as an author, editor, or publisher. He is the co-creator, editor, and publisher of the Eat This, Not That! series, and has published such titles as *Wheat Belly, Zero Belly Diet,* and *The Everygirl's Guide to Diet and Fitness*. He is the author of *The New American Diet, The Men's Health Diet,* and *The Women's Health Diet,* and he is the coauthor, with David Zinczenko, of *Zero Sugar Diet* and, with Danica Patrick, of *Pretty Intense*. Perrine is the co-creator and co–executive producer of *Better Man*, a nationally syndicated health and wellness TV show for men. The former editor-in-chief of *Best Life* and editorial creative director of *Men's Health*, he has appeared as a nutrition and weight-loss expert on a wide variety of programs including *Dr. Oz, Today, Good Morning America, The Early Show,* and the *700 Club*. He lives in Westport, Connecticut. Follow him on Twitter @EatWellNYC.

Heidi Skolnik is a nutritionist and exercise scientist whose career spans clinical nutrition, public education, and performance nutrition with professional athletes and Broadway stars. She has appeared extensively on national TV including the *Today Show, Live! With Kelly and Michael, Good Morning America, The Early Show, Dr. Oz*, and the Food Network. She oversees Performance Nutrition at the Juilliard School and School of American Ballet and sees clients at the Women's Sports Medicine Center at the Hospital for Special Surgery. Skolnik has served as team nutritionist for the New York Giants, New York Knicks, and New York Mets. She sits on the advisory board of the National Menopause Foundation and served as a board member of the National Osteoporosis Foundation for ten years. She is the author of *Grill Yourself Skinny* and is the creator of *The Athlete Triad Playbooks*, a training manual for exercise professionals. She is coauthor of *Nutrient Timing for Peak Performance* and *The Reverse Diet*. She lives in New Jersey.

AARP is the nation's largest nonprofit, nonpartisan organization dedicated to empowering people fifty and older to choose how they live as they age. With a nationwide presence, AARP strengthens communities and advocates for what matters most to families: health security, financial stability, and personal fulfillment. AARP also produces the nation's largest circulation publications, *AARP The Magazine* and the *AARP Bulletin*, which reach AARP's 38 million members.